Quick & Easy
Dosage Calculations

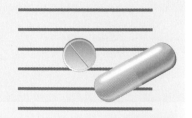

Quick & Easy
Dosage Calculations:
Using Dimensional Analysis

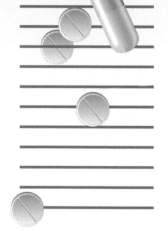

Christina Wu Nasrawi, PhD, MSN, FNP
President
Good Neighbor Medical Clinic
Fresno, CA

Formerly, Assistant Professor
Department of Chemistry
California State University, Fresno
Fresno, CA

Judith A. Allender, RN, C, MSN, EdD
Professor
Department of Nursing
School of Health & Human Services
California State University, Fresno
Fresno, CA

W.B. SAUNDERS COMPANY
A Division of Harcourt Brace & Company
Philadelphia   London   Toronto   Montreal   Sydney   Tokyo

W.B. SAUNDERS COMPANY
A Division of Harcourt Brace & Company

The Curtis Center
Independence Square West
Philadelphia, Pennsylvania 19106

Library of Congress Cataloging-in-Publication Data

Nasrawi, Christina Wu.
Quick and easy dosage calculations/Christina Wu Nasrawi, Judith
A. Allender.—1st ed.

p.   cm.

Includes bibliographical references and index.

ISBN 0–7216–7133–0

1. Pharmaceutical arithmetic.   I. Allender, Judith Ann.   II. Title.
  [DNLM: 1. Pharmaceutical Preparations—administration & dosage nurses' instruction.
  2. Mathematics nurses' instruction.   QV 748 N264q 1999]

RS57.N36 1999   615′.14—dc21

DNLM/DLC   98–24851

QUICK & EASY DOSAGE CALCULATIONS: Using Dimensional Analysis   ISBN 0–7216–7133–0

Printed in the United States of America.

Last digit is the print number: 9   8   7   6   5   4   3   2   1

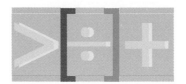

Reviewers

Sharon Beasley, MSN, RN
Rend Lake College
Ina, Illinois

Rosemarie Blume, MA, RN
Professor, Nursing Department
County College of Morris
Randolph, New Jersey

Jane D. Brannan, EdD, RN
Kennesaw State University
Kennesaw, Georgia

Barbara A. Ihrke, MS, RN
Assistant Professor
Indiana Wesleyan University
Marion, Indiana

Pauline M. Green, PhD, RN
College of Nursing
Howard University
Washington, District of Columbia

Anita L. Thorne, MA, RN
Clinical Associate Professor
College of Nursing
Arizona State University
Tempe, Arizona

Patricia A. Lange-Otsuka, MSN, RN,
    CS, CCRN
Hawaii Pacific University
Kaneohe, Hawaii

Rebecca Sue Poore, RN, BSN,
    CCRN
American Transitional Hospital
Tulsa, Oklahoma

Dorothy Ann Walker, MSN, RN
Indiana University Kokomo
Kokomo, Indiana

Carolyn Johnson Wyss, MSN, RN
Walters State Community College
Morristown, Tennessee

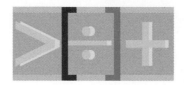

Student Reviewers

Clayton R. Allen
Oregon Health Sciences University
Portland, Oregon

Melissa L. Curtis
SUNY Health Science Center
Syracuse, New York

Dawn Crews
Winston Salem State University
Winston Salem, North Carolina

Lee Ann Grogan
Cincinnati State Technical &
   Community College
College of Mount St. Joseph
Cincinnati, Ohio

Jessica Hughes
Mesa State College
Grand Junction, Colorado

Leslie Jo Mitchell
George Mason University
Fairfax, Virginia

Susan L. Ryan
Rutgers, The State University of
   New Jersey
Newark, New Jersey

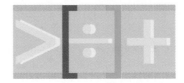

Preface

The intent of this book is to introduce the student to a method of calculating medication dosages that eliminates errors and saves time. Dimensional analysis is a calculation concept that has been used routinely and successfully in chemistry and is coming into use in pharmacy and nursing. The dimensional analysis approach to dosage calculation simplifies the seemingly complex nature of deciding the correct medication dose for a client when solutions come in large volumes or must be mixed with other solutions, or when the medication does not come in the dose ordered by the primary care provider.

Over the years, educators have discovered that students, especially adults, learn best with self-paced materials. Presenting new information in a format that allows students to absorb the material at their own pace reinforces learned concepts throughout each chapter. This format uses a variety of presentation styles, which also enhances learning.

Quick & Easy Dosage Calculations progresses from simple to complex, a format for learning that is basic in most educational settings. So as not to confuse the student who is new to this method, we introduce only the basic mathematical concepts that the student needs in order to be successful with the dimensional analysis approach. This book is not intended to replace basic textbooks in mathematics, pharmacology, or nursing fundamentals. We envision its being used throughout a nursing program as a supplement to standard nursing textbooks while the student learns to administer medications in increasingly complex situations.

Students can use dimensional analysis successfully if they have an understanding of basic mathematics, including addition, subtraction, multiplication, division, fractions, ratios, decimals, and household, metric, and apothecary measurements. Students enter the nursing program with basic mathematical skills acquired in previous settings. This book begins with a review of the particular skills needed to use dimensional analysis.

Organization

The organization of the book includes three units. Unit I begins with two chapters that review basic mathematical calculations and principles of safe medication administration. Chapter 3 introduces the steps of the dimensional analysis process. Beginning with Chapter 4, dimensional analysis is used to calculate medications that students commonly give early in their educational experience; the focus is on oral, topical, and rectal routes of administration. The following chapters continue with increasingly complex medication administration situations, including intradermal, subcutaneous, intramuscular, and intravenous routes of administration.

In Unit II, we introduce special populations, settings, and medications. These chapters follow the simple-to-complex nature of client needs that is typical in nursing programs. This approach makes the book useful for both faculty and students throughout the nursing curriculum.

The chapters of the book are formatted in a similar manner. Within the body of the chapter, we explain specific medications and routes of administration appropriate to the population or setting presented. Each chapter concludes with a group of problem sets for practice; the correct answers are included. We provide the solutions for these problems in the Instructor's Manual.

Features

A helpful addition to this book is the use of margin notes interjected appropriately and accompanied by symbols that identify the type of important information provided. Four symbols are used in the margin notes throughout the text:

A key ♀ indicates essential principles of mathematical calculation that are basic to safe medication administration.

A traffic light ▮ is a warning that indicates critical or fundamental information.

A pearl ◐ alerts the reader to helpful information gathered from clinical experience.

A magnifying glass ♀ gives hints for solving a dosage calculation or a problem of medication administration.

These symbols offer the reader the kinds of information that instructors often share with students, based upon years of clinical practice, tips from staff nurses or nurse preceptors, and issues not routinely found in textbooks. The rationale for the information in these margin notes is supplied at the same point in the chapter.

The reader may notice that the structure of each page is unique. The pages are designed with a wide margin along the outer side of the book. A vertical line separates the margin from the key content. Along the outer margin, the reader will find the margin notes and symbols referred to previously. The reader will also find correct answers for the pretests, mini-quizzes, and problem sets in each chapter. Using the flap of the book cover, the reader can conceal the answers in this column while working on the problem. Then, the reader can uncover the margin and compare the answers. The extra room in the margin also allows space for students to work out the problems on their own. Learning is continuously reinforced in each chapter.

Comprehensive Problem Set Examination

The book concludes with Unit III, which consists of a group of practice problems for final review of the dosage calculations. Odd-numbered answers follow the questions. Even-numbered answers appear in the Instructor's Manual. The level of difficulty of the problems progresses from simple to complex. The problem sets in Chapters 4 through 12 can be issued as one examination, or they can be combined with the final chapter as a comprehensive examination to test the students' competence in using dimensional analysis. Solutions for the problems in the textbook, including the comprehensive examination, are provided in the Instructor's Manual. The solutions show students how to work through each problem. Instructors may choose to photocopy the solutions for their students so they can see how to solve each problem.

We hope that faculty and students who use *Quick & Easy Dosage Calculations* find it to be the *pearl* they have been looking for to assist them in mastering the *key* concepts and medication calculations necessary for providing safe care to clients, whether their medication needs are simple or complex.

Christina W. Nasrawi
Judith A. Allender

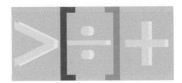

Acknowledgments

To the reviewers, thank you all for providing the constructive insights that help present the concept of dimensional analysis.

To Cynthia Berg, because your vision made this project become a reality.

To Thomas Eoyang, Vice President & Editor-in-Chief, and Maura Connor, Senior Editor, for your insights and faith in this project and for helping to bring it to fruition.

To Victoria Legnini, Editorial Assistant, and Stephanie Klein, formerly of W.B. Saunders Company, for keeping all the wheels in motion throughout the developmental process.

To Mary Reinwald, Copy Editor, and Linda Garber, Senior Production Manager, a big thank you for your endless detailed work.

To all of W.B. Saunders Company, we appreciate your support.

To Cynthia Wu, RN, CCRN, thank you for adding realism to the medication dosage questions based on scenarios in critical and intensive care settings; these scenarios add depth to the medication administration for critically ill clients.

To our spouses and families, thank you—we could not have done it without your indulgence.

To all the following companies, thank you for providing medication labels or authorizing the use of labels as a reinforcing tool for learning:

Abana Pharmaceuticals, Inc.
A.H. Robins Company, Inc.
Alcon Laboratories, Inc.
ALPHARMA
Bard Access Systems Inc.
B. Braun Medical, Inc.
Bristol-Myers Squibb Company
    Bristol Laboratories
    Apothecon
Eli Lilly and Company
Endo Pharmaceuticals, Inc.

Purdue Pharma L.P.
Roxane Laboratories, Inc.
SmithKline Beecham
Warner Chilcott, Inc.
Warner-Lambert Company
    Parke-Davis
Wyeth-Ayerst Laboratories (Courtesy of Wyeth-Ayerst Laboratories, Philadelphia, PA)

Christina W. Nasrawi
Judith A. Allender

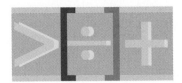

Letter to the Student

Quick & Easy Dosage Calculations is designed to be used throughout your nursing education, and afterward, when as a practicing nurse, you encounter new medication challenges. It contains abbreviations, names, actions, and doses of medications you are currently studying. But how do you figure out *how much* medication to give if the amount available is not the same as that ordered? Dimensional analysis (DA) will help you solve these types of problems. Those of you who have taken courses in chemistry may recognize the concept of dimensional analysis once you read and work through Chapter 2.

Dimensional analysis is relatively new to nursing, and instructors are just beginning to adopt the method in nursing programs across the country. A few institutions have used the method for many years. Once you have mastered dimensional analysis, you may wonder why all nurses do not use it. Probably it is because they were not taught the method in their nursing programs. When you become familiar with dimensional analysis, you will be a resource for others who are struggling with dosage calculations using methods in which right answers can get lost in the many steps required.

Quick & Easy Dosage Calculations is designed to reinforce what you are learning as you go through the book. The correct answers to questions and problems, along with margin notes, constantly guide you in the process of becoming a safe practitioner when administering medications. Pretest questions and answers or a list of facts cue you in to the content of the chapter. At the end of each chapter, you will find a set of problems designed to assess your understanding of the chapter's content, including examples of clients who require simple and complex administration routes; special considerations; community settings, and unique therapies. The organization of the chapters allows you to practice solving problems that are similar to those you encounter in the area of nursing you are currently studying.

At the end of the book, you will find a comprehensive set of problems (followed by correct answers for the odd-numbered problems), that will test your knowledge in all nursing settings. Throughout the text, you will note cartoons depicting some of the dilemmas people get themselves into when they do not calculate dosage problems correctly! Learning all the skills and procedures necessary for becoming a well-prepared and caring nurse will take much of your time in the next few years. Mastering this approach to calculating medication dosages will give you the assurance that you are administering accurate doses as you learn other nursing skills.

Christina W. Nasrawi
Judith A. Allender

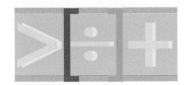

Contents

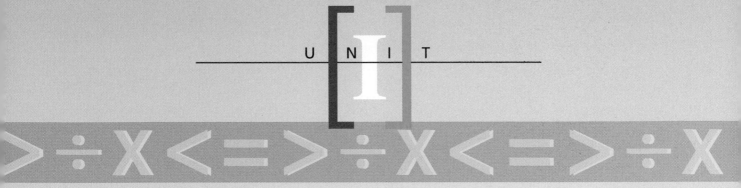

Basic Medication Calculation Using Dimensional Analysis

Unit I, consisting of six chapters, presents the basic concepts of dosage calculation and incorporates dimensional analysis as a tool in dosage calculation. This section begins with the essential mathematical skills that the student needs to calculate dosages by using dimensional analysis and then presents basic safety issues in dosage administration. Chapter 3 is a pivotal chapter. It systematically presents the concept of dimensional analysis. The concept of dimensional analysis is then promptly applied to a variety of medication dosages in Chapters 4 through 6.

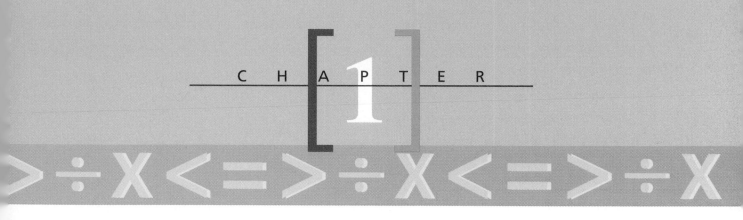

Review of Mathematics and Calculations Used in Dimensional Analysis

INTRODUCTION

At present, the administrators of the National Council Licensure Examination for Registered Nurses (NCLEX-RN) examination do not allow the use of a calculator. The restriction on using a calculator may vary from state to state in the future. Nevertheless, even with a calculator poised in your hand, you still need to know the fundamentals of arithmetic. You need to be proficient in adding, subtracting, multiplying, and dividing numbers. The application of dimensional analysis to dosage calculations requires that you be proficient in multiplication and division.

If you know basic math well enough to multiply and divide, you can skip this chapter and move on to the next chapter. If you have any uncertainty about these skills, please read through this chapter. The goal of this chapter is to provide the tools you need to solve the common mathematical problems found in dosage calculations.

LEARNING OBJECTIVES

By the end of this chapter, you will be able to:

- Demonstrate the multiplication and division processes

- Manipulate decimal places

- Reduce, multiply, and divide fractions

- Convert ratios to fractions and percentages interchangeably

PRETEST: **BASIC MATH**	PRETEST ANSWERS

1. Convert $\dfrac{1}{1000}$ to a decimal.

2. Convert 5% to a decimal.

3. Express 0.025 in ratio format.

4. Convert 1 : 1000 to a percentage.

5. Convert 10% to a fraction.

6. Divide $\dfrac{2}{5}$ by $\dfrac{1}{40}$.

7. Divide 3.8 by 11.5.

8. Express 30% in decimal format.

9. Convert 0.0005 to a percentage.

10. Multiply 1.75 by 0.05.

11. Round 0.867 to the nearest 10th.

12. Round 0.867 to the nearest 100th.

13. Express 0.01 as a fraction.

14. Multiply $\dfrac{3}{4}$ by $\dfrac{8}{21}$.

15. Multiply 0.0011 by 2.8.

16. Divide 2.8 by 0.0011.

17. Convert $\dfrac{1}{3}$ to a ratio.

PRETEST ANSWERS

1. 0.0010

2. 0.050

3. 25 : 1000 or 1 : 40

4. 0.1%

5. $\dfrac{1}{10}$

6. 16

7. 0.3304 = 0.33

8. 0.30

9. 0.05%

10. 0.0875 = 0.088

11. 0.9

12. 0.87

13. $\dfrac{1}{100}$

14. $\dfrac{2}{7}$ = 0.29

15. 0.00308 = 0.0031

16. 2,545.45

17. 1 : 3

MATHEMATICS NEEDED

Decimal Place: Roundup

Dimensional analysis does not devalue the importance of accuracy in math.

A wrong answer remains wrong regardless of the method you use to calculate the medication dosage.

In medication dosage calculation, you will not always get numbers that can be neatly multiplied or divided into whole numbers, so you will need to decide how many decimal places you will need (or want) in your answer. A general rule that you can follow safely with numbers that do not divide to zero residuals is to divide or multiply the numbers and round them to the second decimal place.

If you have numbers that are decimal fractions, that is, not whole numbers, you may need to (if possible) calculate your answer to contain two numbers that are not zeros after the decimal point, e.g., 0.0023, 0.00051. Why? What would you do if you had a number that was a decimal fraction without a whole number, e.g., 0.0001? If you rounded this number to the second decimal place, you would get $0.00 = zero$. In such an instance, you might want to use an exponent (scientific notation), i.e., 1.0×10^{-4}.

To round the third decimal place, that is, if the number at the third decimal place is equal to or greater than five, increase the number in the second decimal place by one. If the number in the third decimal place is less than five, you will keep your answer as is, without the train of numbers after the second decimal place.

The following examples demonstrate significant numbers that are whole and/or decimal fractions.

Always double-check your math.

Make a habit of placing a zero before the decimal point to:
- Clearly emphasize the decimal point
- Decrease the error of misinterpreting decimal fractions for whole numbers

E X A M P L E   1

0.0<u>0</u>00   First decimal place

0.00<u>0</u>0   Second decimal place

0.000<u>0</u>   Third decimal place

E X A M P L E   2

1. Multiply 0.25 by 2.9.
2. Calculate to the second decimal place.

   $0.25 \times 2.9 = 0.725 = 0.73$

The answer contains three decimal places. There are no additional numbers after 0.725; therefore, you can round the third decimal place by increasing the number in the second decimal place by one, that is, 0.725 to 0.73.

E X A M P L E   3

1. Multiply 1.5×2.75.
2. Calculate to the second decimal place.

   $1.5 \times 2.75 = 4.125 = 4.13$

Your answer contains three decimal places, so you can round the 5 in the third decimal place by increasing the number in the second decimal place by one, that is, 4.125 to 4.13. The answer has two decimal places.

When in doubt, round answer to contain two decimal places.

E X A M P L E   4

1. Divide 1.5 by 2.7. Calculate to the second decimal place.

$$\frac{1.5}{2.7} = \underset{\text{Three decimal places}}{0.555} = \underset{\text{Two decimal places}}{0.56}$$

Round the 5 at the third decimal place by increasing the number in the second decimal place by one, that is, $0.555 = 0.56$. Remember, if the number is less than five, you will simply drop it, for example, $0.02044 = 0.02$.

Erroneously moving the decimal point to the left or right by one decimal place causes an error of 10-fold magnitude, that is, the number decreases or increases by a factor of 10, an error that would be significant enough to cause harm to or the death of a client.

In dosage calculations, you cannot follow this rule. Rounding dosage answers depends a great deal on the unit. Here is a short list of instances when a decimal fraction is quite meaningless.

- You cannot have decimal fractions of drops because you cannot split a drop.
- You cannot have decimal fractions of flow rates because infusion pumps are programmed in whole numbers.
- You cannot have decimal fractions of teaspoons other than $0.25 = \frac{1}{4}$, $0.5 = \frac{1}{2}$, and $0.75 = \frac{3}{4}$.
- You cannot have fractions of fluid ounces (fl oz) unless you are willing to convert the fractions into teaspoons or smaller measures.
- You cannot have insulin in a fraction of a unit (U).
- You cannot have decimal fractions of volumes that require syringes of the 20 ml (cc) or larger, because large syringes are not calibrated to measure a fraction of a ml (cc).

It makes no sense to calculate numbers to the third, fourth, fifth, or any subsequent decimal place, if you are not able to measure it. For example, if your answer is 37.74 ml, it is unlikely that you will be able to measure this volume without using three different measuring vessels. So, round it to 38 ml. The exception will be in test situations where the questions are designed to test your ability to keep track of decimals or test your mathematical skills.

In reality, your answer will depend on the scenario of the question. But in a test situation where all the pertinent information is not clearly provided to you, go ahead and round your answers to the second decimal place, or calculate your answers to contain two numbers that are not zeros after the decimal point. In other words, treat a test situation as a math problem, rather than a scenario-based dosage calculation problem.

 For calculated values generated from dosage calculation, keep the decimal fraction in your dosage calculation answer only if you can actually measure it.

 Read the dosage question carefully to determine whether the units (e.g., drops, teaspoons) involved can adequately be measured according to the answer resulting from your calculations.

 If you cannot measure the dosage to the fourth decimal place, what is the use of calculating your answer to the fourth decimal place?

To round a decimal fraction, increase by one the digit to the left of a digit that is equal to or greater than five.

E X A M P L E   5

1.253786 = 1.0	Rounded to whole number
= 1.3	Rounded to one decimal place (10th)
= 1.25	Rounded to two decimal places (100th)
= 1.254	Rounded to three decimal places (1000th)

E X A M P L E   6

0.6329 = 1.0	Rounded to whole number
= 0.6	Rounded to one decimal place (10th)
= 0.63	Rounded to two decimal places (100th)
= 0.633	Rounded to three decimal places (1000th)

E X A M P L E   7

$0.00002074 = 0.0$	Rounded to whole number
$= 0.0$	Rounded to first decimal place
$= 0.00$	Rounded to second decimal place
$= 0.000$	Rounded to third decimal place
$= 0.0000$	Rounded to fourth decimal place
$= 0.00002$	Rounded to fifth decimal place
$= 0.000021$	*Rounded to the sixth decimal place*

$$= 2.1 \times 10^{-5}$$

The scientific notation 10^x represents the number of times you have moved the decimal point, that is, to the right (10^{-x}) or left (10^x).

E X A M P L E   8

Use scientific notation to avoid repetitive zeros after a number or decimal point.

$$1,000,000.0 = 1.0 \times 10^6$$

that is, you have moved the decimal point six places to the left.

$$0.0000001 = 1.0 \times 10^{-7}$$

that is, you have moved the decimal point seven places to the right.

The Multiplication Process

When you multiply numbers with decimals, you need to remember to count the number of decimal places to the right of the decimal point. For example, if there were two numbers to the right of the decimal point, you would have two decimal places; if you had three numbers, you would have three decimal places, and so forth. As for the numbers to the left of the decimal place, you would treat them as you would any whole number.

In multiplying numbers with decimal places, the product (the answer) will always contain the total number of decimal places, that is, the sum of decimal places of the numbers that you are multiplying. For example, in multiplying two numbers, one with two- and one with three-decimal place numbers, the answer will contain five decimal places. The following examples demonstrate the process of multiplying numbers with decimal places.

The answer in multiplication always carries the sum of the decimal places of the two numbers multiplied. For example,

$$\begin{array}{r} \text{2-decimal number} \\ \times\ \text{3-decimal number} \\ \hline \text{5-decimal answer} \end{array}$$

Align the two numbers to the right for multiplication.

E X A M P L E   1

5.72	Two decimal places
$\times 0.002$	Three decimal places
$\overline{1144}$	
000	
$\underline{000}$	
0.01144	Five decimal places

Add a zero to the left of the decimal point to accurately define the decimal point. By doing this, you can prevent numbers from being read erroneously.

Be sure to align the products below each digit that you use to multiply, and add the column for the cumulative product. If necessary, add zeros to the left of the cumulative product to get the total number of decimal places.

It is easier to add, subtract, divide, and multiply with smaller numbers than large ones. Set up your multiplication process so that you are multiplying a difficult number by an easier number.

1. Multiply 5.72 by the 2 in 0.002. Align the product, 1144, under the 2.
2. Multiply by the next number, 0. Align the product, 000, under the 0 to the left of 2.
3. Repeat the process with the next number, also a 0. Align the product, 000, under the 0 to the left of 0.
4. Add the columns of numbers. Product = 01144.
5. Place the decimal point at the fifth place, counting from the far right, that is, 4, 4, 1, 1, 0, then the decimal point.
6. To avoid an error of assumption, write a zero to the left of the decimal to get the answer of 0.01144.

E X A M P L E   2

$$
\begin{array}{rl}
0.012 & \text{Three decimal places} \\
\times\, 0.186 & \text{Three decimal places} \\
\hline
0072 & \\
0096 & \\
0012 & \\
\hline
0.002232 & \text{Six decimal places}
\end{array}
$$

1. Multiply 0.012 by 6 = 0072. Align the product, 0072, under the number 6.
2. Multiply 0.012 by 8 = 0096. Align the product, 0096, under the number 8.
3. Multiply 0.012 by 1 = 0012. Align the product, 0012, under the number 1.
4. Add the columns. Sum = 002232.
5. Place the decimal point to the left of the last 0.
6. Your answer is 0.002232.

Let's look at this problem again. You may think that it will be easier to multiply 0.186 by 0.012. Certainly, it can also be done that way!

$$
\begin{array}{r}
0.186 \\
\times\, 0.012 \\
\hline
0372 \\
0186 \\
0000 \\
\hline
0.002232
\end{array}
$$

Look for opportunities to multiply with smaller numbers. The answer is the same. In this case, it is by far easier to multiply numbers with 1 and 2 than the larger numbers of 6 and 8, as in the previous setup. In mathematics, whenever you have a chance, look for ways of carrying out the needed calculations using smaller numbers in the problem set. For example, if you need to multiply 250 × 2, it is far easier to conceptualize the doubling of 250 than increasing 2 by 250 fold.

E X A M P L E   3

```
    52.89        Two decimal places
 ×  4.51         Two decimal places
   5289
  26445
  21156
 238.5339        Four decimal places
```

1. Multiply 5289 by 1 = 5289. Align the product, 5289, under the number 1.
2. Multiply 5289 by 5. Product = 26445. Align 26445 under the number 5.
3. Multiply 5289 by 4. Product = 21156. Align 21156 under the number 4.
4. Add the columns. The sum is 2385339.
5. To place the decimal point, start your place count from the far right, that is, 9, 3, 3, 5.
6. Place the decimal point at the fourth place, between 8 and 5, to get your answer. Product = 238.5339.

M I N I   Q U I Z

How many decimal places would you have in the product of example 3?

Which of the following is easier to do?

a. Multiply 52.89 by 4.51.
b. Multiply 4.51 by 52.89.

Answer: Four decimal places

Answer: a

You only need to multiply with three numbers that are smaller numerically and therefore easier to handle.

The Division Process: Fractions and Decimals

You can write the two numbers you need to divide in a fraction format. The fraction format consists of two numbers separated by a line. The number at the top is called the numerator (N), and the bottom number is called the denominator (D).

When dividing the numerator by the denominator, you can convert a fraction into a whole number with or without decimal places. You need to know how to move the decimal point in the process of dividing numbers.

In a fraction setup, you can make the numbers larger or smaller by a factor of 10 by moving the decimal point to either the left (smaller) or the right (larger). You need to apply the process of inflation or deflation to both the top (numerator) and the bottom (denominator). They must be moved the same number of times. After all, you do not want to change the value of the fraction. You just want to make it smaller or larger so you can better handle it in the calculation process.

The following examples demonstrate how you can inflate or deflate a fraction to help you solve problems.

 Use either fractions or decimals, whichever makes you more comfortable.

 Move the decimal point to the left or right to decrease or increase numbers by factors of 10, to make numbers easier to conceptualize and thereby easier to calculate.

 Both halves of a fraction must be treated equally to obtain a correct response.

"ONE OF YOU DID REALLY WELL ON
YOUR MULTIPLICATION TEST!"

You must move the decimal points the same number of places in both the numerator (N) and the denominator (D). If you move the decimal point by two places in the numerator, you must do the same with the decimal point in the denominator.

Manipulating the decimal point allows you to convert numbers for easier handling. The answer remains the same.

E X A M P L E   1

Moving decimals to the right

$$\frac{0.012}{0.5} = \frac{0.12}{5.0} = \frac{1.2}{50} = \frac{12}{500} = 0.024$$

Move the decimals to the right *at the top and bottom* to achieve a desirable fraction. Now, do the division.

E X A M P L E   2

Moving decimals to the right

$$\frac{0.000342}{0.002} = \frac{0.00342}{0.02} = \frac{0.0342}{0.2} = \frac{0.342}{2.0} = 0.171$$

E X A M P L E   3

Moving decimals to the left

$$\frac{134.67}{250} = \frac{13.467}{25} = \frac{1.3467}{2.5} = 0.53868$$

E X A M P L E	4

Moving decimals to the left

$$\frac{5100}{17000} = \frac{510.0}{1700.0} = \frac{51.00}{170.00} = \frac{5.100}{17.000} = 0.3$$

Here are a few examples of long division.

E X A M P L E	5

$$\frac{1}{2} = 0.5$$

Steps:

```
        A        B         C
        0        0.        0.5
     2)1.     2)1.0     2)1.0
                          1 0
                          ___
                            0
```

1. The numerator, 1, becomes the dividend; that is, 1 is placed within the division symbol. Place a decimal point to the right of the dividend (numerator) (Step A).

2. Place a decimal point on the line above (the answer, or quotient). Align the decimal point in the answer directly over the decimal point in the numerator (Step B).

3. The numerator has been inflated by a factor of 10, that is, 1 and 0 = 10 (Step B).

4. Divide 10 by 2.

5. 2 × **5** = 10 (Step C). Place the 5 to the right side of the decimal point in the answer.

6. Subtract 10 from the numerator (Step C). The residual is 0. There is nothing left to divide.

7. Your answer is 0.5.

E X A M P L E	6

$$\frac{1}{1000} = 0.001$$

Steps:

```
          A             B             C              D
          0.            0.0           0.00           0.001
   1000)1.0      1000)1.00     1000)1.000     1000)1.000
                                                     1000
                                                     ____
                                                        0
```

1. Place a decimal point on the answer line (quotient) and add a zero to the right of the numerator (dividend) to get 1.0 (Step A). Remember to write a zero to the left of the decimal point.

2. Place the decimal point directly above the decimal point in the numerator (Step A).

Subsequent addition of zeros after the decimal point will further inflate or increase the numerator by a factor of 10 with each zero added.

Remember to write the decimal point (and the zeros) in your answer as you inflate the numerator for division by a factor of 10 with each zero.

To avoid an error, remember to write down each step as you carry out the division process.

Each decimal place error results in an error of a 10-fold increase or decrease in medication dosage calculation and is *dangerous* (if not deadly).

3. Add zero to the right of the decimal point on the answer line and add a zero to the numerator to get 1.00 (Step B).

4. Add another zero to the right of the zero you have just finished adding to the answer line, and add another zero to the numerator to get 1.000 (Step C).

5. Now the numerator (dividend) is large enough to be divided by the denominator (divisor). Divide 1.000 by 1000 to get **1** (the decimal point in the numerator is ignored). Place the 1 to the right of the two zeros on the answer line to get 0.001 (Step D).

6. Subtract 1000 from the numerator. The remainder is 0. There is nothing left to divide.

7. Your answer is 0.001.

 Always double-check your math by repeating the calculation process.

E X A M P L E   7

$$\frac{17}{25} = 0.68$$

Steps: A   B   C

$$\begin{array}{r} 0. \\ 25\overline{)17.0} \end{array} \qquad \begin{array}{r} 0.6 \\ 25\overline{)17.00} \\ 150 \\ \hline 200 \end{array} \qquad \begin{array}{r} 0.68 \\ 25\overline{)17.00} \\ 150 \\ \hline 200 \\ 200 \\ \hline 0 \end{array}$$

1. Place a decimal point on the answer line and add a zero to the right of 17 to get 17.0 (Step A). Remember to place a zero to the left of the decimal point on the answer line.

2. Place the decimal point in the answer directly above the decimal point of numerator, or dividend (Step A).

3. $25 \times \mathbf{6} = 150$. Subtract 150 from the numerator. The remainder is 20 (Step B).

4. Place the 6 on the right side of the decimal point in the answer (Step B).

5. Automatically add a zero to your remainder to inflate the remainder from 20 to 200 (Step B).

6. $25 \times \mathbf{8} = 200$. Subtract 200 from 200. The remainder is zero. There is nothing left to divide (Step C).

7. Place the 8 to the right of 6 to get 0.68 (Step C).

8. Your answer is 0.68 (Step C).

Fractions: Reduction and Multiplication

 Reducing fractions through cancellation/division of numerators and denominators often yields numbers small enough for easy manipulation.

In multiplying fractions, you can use two techniques to get to your answer. With the first technique, you multiply all the numerators (N) and then multiply all the denominators (D). Your final step will consist of reducing the composite fraction (N/D) down to the lowest usable number and dividing the numerator by the denominator.

The second technique consists of reducing the individual fractions down to manageable numbers and then multiplying the remaining numerators and denominators. Choose whichever technique is easier for you.

To reduce a fraction or a row of fractions, you can divide both the numerator and the denominator by the same number. You can also cancel numbers that are the same in both the numerator and the denominator.

E X A M P L E   1

$$\frac{1}{2} \times \frac{2}{5} = \frac{2}{\cancel{10}} = \frac{1}{5}$$

1. Multiply the numbers on the top: $1 \times 2 = 2$.
2. Multiply the numbers on the bottom: $2 \times 5 = 10$.
3. The fraction $\frac{1}{2}$ can be reduced to 1 by dividing both the top and the bottom by the same number.
4. In this case, we divide the top and bottom by 2, or,

$$\frac{1}{\cancel{2}} \times \frac{\cancel{2}}{5} = \frac{1}{5}$$

1. Cancel numbers that are the same on the top and bottom, that is, 2.
2. Multiply what is left on the top and bottom.

E X A M P L E   2

$$\frac{3}{8} \times \frac{1}{3} = \frac{3}{\cancel{24}} = \frac{1}{8}$$

1. Multiply the top numbers: $3 \times 1 = 3$.
2. Multiply the bottom numbers: $8 \times 3 = 24$.
3. Reduce the fraction by dividing the top and bottom numbers by 3, or

$$\frac{3}{8} \times \frac{1}{3} = \frac{1}{8}$$

1. Cancel the numbers that are the same on the top and bottom, that is, 3.
2. Multiply what is left on the top and bottom.

E X A M P L E   3

$$\frac{158}{2.2} \times \frac{1.2}{4.9} \times \frac{35}{1.6} = \frac{6636}{17.248} = 384.74$$

1. Multiply the numerators, $158 \times 1.2 \times 35 = 6636$.
2. Multiply the denominators, $2.2 \times 4.9 \times 1.6 = 17.248$.
3. Divide 6636 by 17.248 (Good luck!).
4. The answer is 384.74.

Try this instead:

$$\frac{\overset{79}{\cancel{158}}}{\underset{1.1}{\cancel{2.2}}} \times \frac{\overset{0.3}{\cancel{1.2}}}{\underset{0.7}{\cancel{4.9}}} \times \frac{\overset{5}{\cancel{35}}}{\underset{0.4}{\cancel{1.6}}} = \frac{118.5}{0.308} = 384.74$$

 Reduce large numbers with a common denominator; that is, reduce 2 and 10 by 2 to get 1 and 5.

 If you decide to reduce numbers in fractions, remember to reduce both the numerator and the denominator.

 Look for numbers to cancel that are the same in the numerator and denominator.

 To avoid introduction of error, keep track of what you have cancelled and what is left for multiplication and division.

1. Reduce 2.2 and 158 by 2 to get 1.1 and 79.
2. Reduce 4.9 and 35 by 7 to get 0.7 and 5.
3. Reduce 1.6 and 1.2 by 4 to get 0.4 and 0.3.
4. Multiply what's left in the numerator, $79 \times 0.3 \times 5 = 118.5$.
5. Multiply what's left in the denominator, $1.1 \times 0.7 \times 0.4 = 0.308$.
6. Divide 118.5 by $0.308 = 384.7402$. To divide 118.5 by 0.308, convert 0.308 to 308 and 118.5 to 118500, by moving the decimal point three places to the right.

```
            384.7402
308)118500.00
    924
    2610
    2464
     1460
     1232
      2280
      2156
       1240
       1232
        800
        616   ← Stop here!
        184   There are already 2 decimal places.
```

Please, no more!

7. Have your answer contain two decimal places; that is, 384.74.

Fractions: Division

To divide fractions, first you need to invert the fraction (flip it over) that serves as the denominator. Then you simply multiply the two fractions for your answer.

Dividing a whole number divided by a fraction:

$$\frac{C}{\frac{A}{B}} = \frac{C}{A} \times B = C \times \frac{B}{A}$$

C = the whole number.
A/B = fraction.

You can either:

• Divide A by B, then use the answer to divide C, or
• Flip the fraction A/B, to B/A, then multiply the inverted fraction with the whole number C.

Dividing Two Fractions

E X A M P L E   1

$$\frac{\dfrac{3}{5}}{\dfrac{2}{9}} = \frac{3}{5} \times \frac{9}{2} \quad \substack{\text{Inverted} \\ \text{denominator}} \quad = \frac{27}{10} = 2.7$$

1. Flip the denominator fraction that is, $\dfrac{2}{9}$ to $\dfrac{9}{2}$.

2. Multiply $\dfrac{3}{5}$ by $\dfrac{9}{2}$.

3. Multiply the numerators, $3 \times 9 = 27$, and the denominators, $5 \times 2 = 10$.

4. Divide 27 by 10. Answer is 2.7.

$$\frac{\dfrac{C}{D}}{\dfrac{A}{B}} = \frac{C}{D} \times \frac{B}{A}$$

C/D = numerator fraction.

A/B = denominator fraction.

You can divide a fraction with another fraction by either of two methods:

- Individually solving each fraction and then dividing the two answers, or

1. Flipping the denominator fraction upside down, so that A/B becomes B/A, and

2. Then multiplying the two fractions, that is, C/D × B/A.

E X A M P L E   2

$$\frac{\dfrac{15}{7}}{\dfrac{2.7}{0.24}} = \frac{\overset{5.0}{\cancel{15}}}{7} \times \frac{\overset{0.08}{\cancel{0.24}}}{\underset{\underset{0.3}{0.9}}{\cancel{2.7}}} = \frac{0.40}{2.1} = 0.190 = 0.19$$

1. Flip the denominator fraction to $\dfrac{0.24}{2.7}$.

2. Multiply $\dfrac{15}{7}$ by $\dfrac{0.24}{2.7}$.

3. First, reduce 15 and 2.7 by a factor of 3 to get 5.0 and 0.9.

4. Next, reduce 0.24 and 0.9 by a factor of 3.

5. Then, multiply the remaining numerators, $5 \times 0.08 = 0.40$, and the denominator, that is, $7 \times 0.3 = 2.1$.

6. Finally, divide 0.4 by 2.1. Answer = 0.190, = 0.19, as follows:

Step:	A	B	C	D
	0.	0.1	0.19	0.1904
	2.1$\overline{)0.40}$	2.1$\overline{)0.400}$	2.1$\overline{)0.400}$	2.1$\overline{)0.400}$
		21	21	21
		190	190	190
			189	189
			10	100
				84
				16

1. Put a decimal point on the answer line and add a zero to the right of 0.4 to inflate it to 0.40 (Step A). Remember to place a zero to the left of the decimal point on the answer line to clearly indicate a decimal fraction.
2. Divide 0.40 by 0.21 (ignore decimal points), so 21 × *1* = 21. Subtract 21 from 40. The residual is 19 (step B).
3. Place 1 to the right side of the decimal point on the answer line (Step B).
4. Placement of 1 in the answer allows automatic inflation of the residual from 19 to 190 (Step B).
5. Divide 190 by 21, so 21 × *9* = 189. Subtract 189 from 190. The remainder is 1.
6. On the answer line, place 9 to the right of 0.1 to get 0.19 (Step C). The remainder gains a zero from 1 to 10.

 Don't forget to *invert, or flip, the fraction that is doing the dividing* (denominator fraction) upside down before you start multiplying.

The key to division and multiplication of numbers lies in your mastery of the multiplication tables.

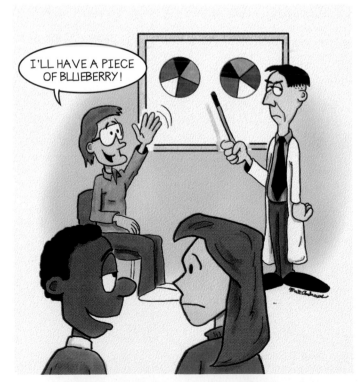

"I THINK GILBERT MISSED THE CONCEPT OF PIE CHARTS!"

7. You need to add a zero to your answer to inflate 10 to 100. (Step D). Divide 100 by 21, so that 21 × *4* = 84. Subtract 84 from 100. The remainder is 16.
8. Place 4 to the right of 0.190 to get 0.1904.
9. You now have an answer with four decimal places and with four significant numbers. To keep the answer at two decimal places, simply drop the last two. Your answer is 0.19.

Percentages and Ratios

Percentage is just another format used to present a fraction with a denominator that is always 100. Percentage is used quite frequently because most people can grasp the concept of proportions based on 100 parts.

 Stop the division process when it becomes abundantly clear that the third decimal place will not make a difference to the second decimal place, that is, you cannot get a number equal to or greater than five to round.

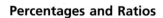

$$3\% = 3 \text{ parts out of } 100 = \frac{3}{100} = 0.03$$

1. Convert a percentage to a fraction by dividing by 100.
2. Convert a fraction to a decimal by dividing 3 by 100. Answer = 0.03.

 You can convert any number into a fraction by dividing it by 1.

 Percentage = parts per hundred, that is, 3% = 3 parts per 100, which is equal to 3/100 in a fraction format.

E X A M P L E   2

$$98.5\% = 98.5 \text{ parts per } 100 = \frac{98.5}{100} = 0.985$$

 Other commonly used ratios include parts per thousand (ppt), parts per million (ppm), parts per billion (ppb), and so forth.

E X A M P L E   3

$$7.5\% = 7.5 \text{ parts per } 100 = \frac{7.5}{100} = 0.075$$

 The first number of the ratio always serves as the numerator of a fraction, that is, first is top and top is first.

Ratios are proportions or fractions written in a different way. Instead of a line between two numbers, we use a symbol that looks every bit like a colon, that is, (:). A ratio between two numbers, a and b, can be written as a:b. Whenever you see two numbers that are separated by these two dots, you can safely rewrite them in a fraction format where the first number is the numerator, and the second the denominator.

 In dosage calculation, ratio represents proportion between the numerator and the denominator, that is, parts of numerator per parts of denominator.

E X A M P L E   4

$$1:2 = 1 \text{ part per 2 parts} = \tfrac{1}{2} = 0.5 = 50\%$$

1. The first number of a ratio is equal to the numerator.
2. The number after the colon (:) is measured in proportion to the first number, that is, 1 part of numerator per 2 parts of denominator $= \tfrac{1}{2}$.
3. You can convert $\tfrac{1}{2}$ to a decimal and a percentage.

Answer: 1 part per million.

Explain the ratio $1 : 1,000,000$.

E X A M P L E 5

$$1 : 10 = \frac{1}{10}$$

1. $1 : 10$ can be rewritten as a fraction.
2. The first number, 1, becomes the numerator, and the second the denominator.
3. Convert a fraction to a decimal by dividing 1 by 10. Answer = 0.1.
4. Convert a decimal to a fraction by dividing by 1. Answer = $\frac{0.1}{1}$.
5. Multiply by 100 to convert to a percentage. Product = 10%.

Therefore, you can rewrite $1 : 10$ as the following:

$$1 : 10 = \frac{1}{10} = 0.1 = \frac{0.1}{1} \times 100 = 10\%$$

E X A M P L E 6

$$1.5 : 1000 = \frac{1.5}{1000}$$

1. The first number, 1.5, is the numerator, and the second is the denominator.
2. Divide 1.5 by 1000 to convert the ratio or fraction to a decimal. Answer = 0.0015
3. Multiply the fraction by 100 to rewrite it as a percentage. Product = 0.15%

Therefore, you can rewrite $1.5 : 1000$ as the following:

$$1.5 : 1000 = \frac{1.5}{1000} = 0.0015 = \frac{0.0015}{1} \times 100 = 0.15\%$$

 Fractions, ratios, and percentages are ways that you can write numbers. Therefore, you can convert numbers from one format to another by simple mathematical manipulations.

Rewrite 5 parts per billion in a ratio format and in a fraction format.

Answer: $5 : 1,000,000,000$, or

$$\frac{5}{1,000,000,000}$$

Scientific Notation

Scientific notation is just another way of writing numbers for easier handling. It consists of two parts:

1. A whole number with or without decimals (frequently up to two decimal places), and

 Scientific notation helps you manage numbers that are excessively large to write: millions, billions, or numbers with decimal places greater than 4.

2. The number 10, with either positive or negative powers, that is, 10^9, 10^{-3}, 10^{-6}. The powers represent the number of factors in multiples of 10.

E X A M P L E   1

$2.56 \times 10^{-12} = 0.000,000,000,00256$

M I N I   Q U I Z

Convert 8.3 parts per million into decimal and scientific notation formats.

Answer: 0.0000083, or 8.3 $\times$ 10^{-6}

E X A M P L E   2

$7.91 \times 10^{10} = 79,100,000,000$

 Rewrite a scientific notation number as a decimal by moving the decimal point to the left or to the right.

Chapter Summary

Several different examples have demonstrated to you the mathematical skills necessary to carry out dosage calculations. Additionally, the different ways of describing numbers in the format of ratios, percentages, fractions, and decimals have been reviewed. The mastery of addition, subtraction, multiplication, and division is necessary to effectively calculate dosage problems. The use of both metric (decimals), and arithmetic systems (ratios, fractions, percentages), in dosage problems necessitates that you have a clear understanding of these operatives. Therefore, if you are still having problems with the basic mathematics, please review this chapter again before you proceed to the next.

PROBLEM SET	PROBLEM SET ANSWERS

Multiplication and Division Processes.

1. $500 \times \dfrac{1}{8} =$

1. 62.50

2. $1000 \times 0.0025 =$

2. 2.50

PROBLEM SET	PROBLEM SET ANSWERS
3. $40 \times 20 =$	3. 800
4. $0.25 \times 15 =$	4. 3.75
5. $125 \times \dfrac{1}{2.2} =$	5. 56.82
6. $1000 \times \dfrac{1}{24} =$	6. 41.67

Manipulation of Decimal Places.

1. 0.00256 to three decimal places	1. 0.003
2. 1.27 to a whole number	2. 1.0
3. 9.98 to a whole number	3. 10.0
4. 2.967 to two decimal places	4. 2.97
5. 7.53 to one decimal place	5. 7.5

PROBLEM SET	PROBLEM SET ANSWERS

6. 3.125 to two decimal places

6. 3.13

Reduce, Multiply, and Divide Fractions.

1. $\dfrac{1.6}{1.3} \times \dfrac{2.6}{7} \times \dfrac{1}{4} =$

1. $0.114 = 0.11$

2. $\dfrac{3}{7} \times \dfrac{12.9}{2.1} \times \dfrac{2}{9} =$

2. $0.585 = 0.59$

3. $\dfrac{\frac{4}{1}}{\frac{7}{5}} \times 1.25 =$

3. $3.571 = 3.57$

4. $\dfrac{89}{2.2} \times \dfrac{25}{3} =$

4. $337.121 = 337.12$

5. $\dfrac{25}{4} \times \dfrac{3}{100} \times \dfrac{1}{30} \times 4 =$

5. 0.025

6. $\dfrac{38.2}{2.2} \times 3.0 \times \dfrac{0.6}{15} =$

6. $2.0836 = 2.08$

PROBLEM SET	PROBLEM SET ANSWERS

7. $\dfrac{1000}{\dfrac{1}{15}} \times \dfrac{1}{60} =$

7. 250

Convert Ratios to Fractions and Percentages Interchangeably.

1. 50% =   :   = ——

1. 1:2, $\dfrac{1}{2}$

2. 5% =   :   = ——

2. 1:20, $\dfrac{1}{20}$

3. $\dfrac{2}{3}$ = % =   :

3. 66.67%,   2:3

4. 10% =   :   = ——

4. 1:10, $\dfrac{1}{10}$

5. 0.9% =   :   = ——

5. 0.9:100 or 9:1000, $\dfrac{0.9}{100}$ or $\dfrac{9}{1000}$

6. 1 = % = ——

6. 100%, $\dfrac{1}{1}$

2

Safety Principles and Practices With Medication Administration

INTRODUCTION

In this chapter, basic concepts in dosage administration will be discussed. Principles of pharmacology will not be discussed in great detail. Numerous pharmacology textbooks discuss issues concerning safe administration of medication and techniques of administration. This chapter will give you the absolute basics of administering medication safely to your patients.

LEARNING OBJECTIVES

By the end of this chapter, you will be able to:

- List the basic safety principles regarding dosage administration by identifying the three checks and the five rights

- Discuss implications of the nursing process in dosage administration

- Highlight the right to refuse treatment under the patient's bill of rights

- Discuss issues concerning medications with similar spelling that look alike on written orders

Continued

- Discuss issues concerning medications that sound similar depending on how they are pronounced
- Interpret abbreviations found in medication orders and patients' charts
- Interpret medication dosage orders
- Recognize the importance of reading drug labels
- Interpret dosage information from drug labels

BASIC SAFETY CONCEPTS IN DOSAGE ADMINISTRATION

 Patient safety is a nurse's first priority.

 Once administered, you cannot take back a medication.

 The order is the originating point of a dosage.

 Make sure the order is written legibly and the content is clearly understood.

 Ask for the spelling of the medication if it is unclear. Confirm drug, dosage, and schedule of dosage by reading the order back to the provider.

 Be your patient's advocate.

 All nurses start as novices and gradually advance through experience and continuing education to gain knowledge and skills.

The issue of safety is an integral part of medication administration. In addition to improper use and/or confusing abbreviations, medication errors are frequently linked to the wrong patient, drug, dosage, route of administration, and/or time of administration. Unfortunately, medication errors do not stop with what has been discussed so far. Here is a short list of things that could go wrong in dosage calculation and medication administration.

1. The written orders are not very clearly stated or are illegibly written.
2. The telephone order was taken incorrectly.
3. The written order was transcribed incorrectly.
4. More than one label is on the drug delivered to you.
5. The wrong equipment is used to administer medication.
6. The equipment malfunctions or is improperly used.
7. Medications are improperly handled and/or stored.
8. Medication is given to a patient with a contraindicating condition.
9. Protocol is not understood or is violated.

If you cannot understand the order, it is your responsibility to double-check. If a new order is not clear, the best thing to do is to get clarification from the doctor or provider (advanced-practice nurse, physician assistant, licensed psychologist) who ordered it. If the order is an existing one, a fellow nurse who has taken care of this particular patient on previous shifts or the pharmacist can help.

As a nurse, your primary directive is to provide nursing care to patients by serving as a patient advocate (one who speaks up for another). Medication administration is only a part of the nursing care that you are providing. Consider the importance of your role as a nurse—your patient's health and/or life may depend on your skillful caregiving, including proper medication calculation and administration.

Education received in nursing programs gives beginning students the knowledge essential for providing safe and basic nursing care. As your nursing career matures, particularly in the area of specialty that you will be involved in, you will gain additional knowledge and the skills necessary for providing care to patients in more complex situations that require advanced decision-making.

Medications—How Supplied?

The provider writes medication orders on the patient's chart. Also, the provider can give a verbal order to the nurse. The nurse transcribes the order and sends it along to the pharmacy to get the order filled. Depending on the site and/or type of institution, the pharmacy uses different methods to distribute medication to the patients.

 The pharmacy supplies all medications ordered, including IV solutions.

- Individual prescription—pharmacy fills the prescription(s) in individual medication vials as ordered for each patient.
- Floor-stock system—pharmacy supplies medications kept in a storeroom on the floor in stock bottles. Stock bottles supply the needs of more than one patient.
- Unit-dose system—pharmacy supplies individually packaged medications on a daily (24-hr) basis for patients as ordered. Medications are delivered with an individualized pharmacy administration record for the nurse to document administration of medications.
- Automated system—pharmacy stocks medication in a computerized medication dispenser unit. The nurse uses an identification card to get the medication for administration. The computer automatically records medications dispensed, and information is downloaded on a daily basis.

 Medication orders can be written (in the chart) or verbal (direct or via telephone).

 Look up the rules set by respective institutions on transcription of verbal orders.

 Look up the rules on handling medications that are controlled substances.

Medications are kept secure in designated areas accessible only to nurses. Medications that are considered controlled substances are stored, handled, disposed of, and administered according to regulations established by the US Drug Enforcement Agency and by the respective healthcare institutions.

 The central service supplies syringes, needles, dressings, and other surgical items. Medications are kept secure (locked) in a designated medication box, cupboard, cart, room, etc.

The Three Checks

When you set out to administer the ordered medication dosages to patients, make sure you have reviewed the orders on the respective patients' charts to confirm the order has not been changed. You should also reconcile any differences between the written orders on the chart and the medication list or record provided by the pharmacy.

After making sure that the order is correct, you can set out to administer the medication as ordered. Standing poised to prepare the medication, do the following three checks:

 Check, double-check, and triple-check before you administer the medication dosage.

- ✔ Check the drug or stock bottle against the order or the medication administration record before you count, pour, draw, or mix it; that is, are the medication, route, dosage, and time correct as ordered for the patient?
- ✔ Check the drug against the order after you have poured it and before you put the stock bottle/unit/vial of medication away; that is, are the medication, route, dosage, and time correct as ordered for the patient?
- ✔ Check one last time at the patient's bedside before administering the ordered dosage; that is, are the medication, dosage, time, and route of administration correct for this patient?

 Check medication against the order or pharmacy administration record.

- ✔ Before you pour it
- ✔ After you pour it
- ✔ Before you give it

 Check the spelling of the medication with the provider.

Take time to learn about the medication that you will be administering. If you don't know anything about the drug or are unsure, consult a drug manual. Do not give any medication if you are unfamiliar with it.

A True Story

A public health nurse was opening a case of 144 multidose vials of flu vaccine from a state department of health to administer to waiting lines of senior citizens. Somehow, someone had inadvertently packed one vial of tetanus toxin in the case. The nurse could have been lulled into assuming that all vials in the case were flu vaccine and might have administered a wrong medicine to the waiting seniors. Through careful checking, rechecking, and rechecking again, the error was caught early.

The Five Rights and the Nursing Process

It is important to memorize the five rights concerning dosage administration:

1. Patient—right patient
2. Drug—right drug
3. Dose—right dose
4. Route—right route
5. Time—right time

Nurses apply the nursing process to assess, diagnose, plan, implement, evaluate, and teach. It is within the patient's rights to refuse any treatment. If you individually analyze the three checks and the five rights, along with the nursing process listed in this section, each carries a simple intuitive message; however, on a busy floor with a high patient-to-nurse ratio, the best thing you can do to prevent mishap is to meticulously do the three checks and review the five rights regarding all pertinent nursing processes that constitute the care you administered to your patients.

Even if you do not work in a hospital, you may be employed in a clinic with multiple providers who give you medication orders that may not be written for you to see. You may work in home care where all of your patient's medications are tossed together in a shoebox for you to decipher. Do not be surprised to find prescription medications that have expired. It takes caution to provide safe and effective care efficiently!

Bad handwriting is not an excuse for dosage error.

Use additional items of personal patient data to identify the medication correctly, that is, date of birth, gender, social security number, home address, or telephone number.

Right Patient

Check your patient's name against the identification (ID) wristband printed by the admitting personnel. No matter where you are in the United States, you will be administering medications to non–English-speaking patients. Many of these patients will answer to any name because they do not understand you. Of course, elderly patients may not be able to hear or understand you, while some may be embarrassed to contradict you. Patients with hearing, sight, and/or speech deficits, with or without a decrease in mental acuity, will not be able to respond to your requests. After all, you are the nurse, the person with authority, and "you know what you are doing!"

Keep a current drug manual with you when you are in the clinical laboratory.

Right Drug

Check the order. If you are coming onto a new shift, or returning from several days away from the facility, or even from a lunch break, make sure the order has not been changed in your absence. Sometimes a patient will ask you to give drugs that are the same, one generic, the other a trade name, that is, "I take furosemide in the morning and Lasix at night." Also, don't get lulled into identifying medications by their shape, size, and color.

Right Dose

Check the order. Check the drug dosage. Check your dosage calculation. Again, the order may have changed without your knowledge. Also, the pharmacy may have delivered a different dose of drug since you gave the last dose. The dose you will be administrating is directly dependent on the accuracy of your dosage calculation.

 The pharmacist is a good source of information in clarifying dosage orders and safety issues related to the drug and the patient's diagnosis.

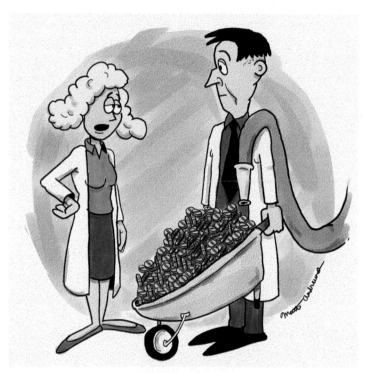

"ARE YOU SURE YOU'RE GIVING THE RIGHT DOSE TO MR. JONES?"

Right Route

Check the order for route of administration. Check the drug, that is, is it the proper dosage form for the route? The pharmacy may have mistakenly sent you an intravenous (IV) dosage instead of the ordered oral form of medication. So, whenever you have any doubt concerning the order, ask for clarification from the provider who placed the order. If the information on the vial or package contradicts the order, ask the pharmacist, "Is it safe to administer this drug according to the order?"

 If you are caring for a patient with multiple IV access, nasogastric tube, or other "lines," be sure to label them to prevent a major life-threatening route error.

Right Time

Check the order. Check the time before you administer the dosage. Document the exact time of your medication administration.

 Be sure there is enough light so you can see what you and your patients are doing.

Check your watch against other timekeeping sources/instruments, for example, clock or radio.

 As a student, you are not allowed to take verbal orders. Your instructor will guide you through such an order.

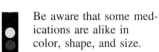 Be aware that some medications are alike in color, shape, and size.

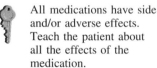 Every medication has a listing of contraindications that define instances when the patient should not be given the medication under question.

 All medications have side and/or adverse effects. Teach the patient about all the effects of the medication.

 Under the patient's bill of rights, the fourth item defines the patient's right to refuse treatment. The courts may overrule a parent's refusal of treatment that could result in the potential death or permanent disability of a child.

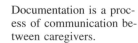 Documentation is a process of communication between caregivers.

Quite often the medications are ordered on a "standing order" basis. With standing orders, you will have about 30 minutes' leeway to administer the dosage as ordered. For example, a standing order of Tylenol ES 1 tab PO q.i.d. p.r.n. fever is the order. You check your administration record and find that the patient received the last dose at 2:30 PM. You can administer the next dose between 8:00 PM and 9:00 PM.

The Nursing Process

After you have checked the five rights discussed previously, you will need to implement the nursing process for safe administration of the dosage ordered for your patient. The nursing process involves cyclical events that require you to assess patients, diagnose conditions, plan and implement care, and evaluate patients, and make adjustments to the plan of care (care plan) accordingly.

This is a summary of the nursing process in dosage administration.

- Assess—patients for subjective and objective expected outcomes related to the disease process and relevant therapeutic agents. Assess the medication's side and/or adverse effects.
- Diagnose—patient's condition by nursing diagnoses established by the North American Nursing Diagnosis Association (NANDA) and by your assessment data and the medication's side and/or adverse effects.
- Plan and Implement—a course of nursing care that reflects your diagnoses.
- Teach—the patient about the disease process, expected outcome from medication related to the disease process, and side and/or adverse effects of medication.
- Evaluate—outcome of implemented plans and make adjustments accordingly, with additional assessments, diagnoses, plans, and patient teaching as part of implementation.

Patient's Bill of Rights, Including Refusal of Treatment

It is recommended that you read the Patient's Bill of Rights (see Appendix) before attempting to provide any form of nursing care to any patient. Additionally, you need to remember that your role as a patient advocate requires that you be aware of and respect the patient's rights.

If your patient refuses treatment, you will need to clearly document the incidences in accordance with the nursing procedure or protocol established at your work site or institution. In addition, documents such as a durable power of attorney and a living will that include "Do Not Resuscitate" (DNR) orders assert the patient's right to choose the quality and quantity of care received. As a patient advocate, you will also need to respect such orders.

Documentation

You will find that most nursing texts contain extensive discussion on the actual process and techniques of recording the patient's progress from admission to discharge. Along with legible penmanship, accuracy and timely documentation of all pertinent information concerning the patient's health condition are crucial parts of safe nursing care.

In a timely fashion document all dosages administered, incidents of side and/or adverse effects related to medication, and outcome. Look for documentation guidelines established by each hospital, clinic, or institution, for example, patient's chart, incident reports, and so forth.

Be objective in your documentation of assessments, for example, 8:00 AM: Edema of lower extremities, pitting, $\frac{2\pm}{4}$ bilaterally, from feet to 2″ below knees; 10:00 AM: Edema of lower extremities, pitting, $\frac{2\pm}{4}$ bilaterally, from feet to 4″ above ankles. Avoid using subjective terms in your documentation, for example, "The patient's legs were pretty swollen earlier and look worse now."

We shall be discussing use of abbreviations in the latter part of this chapter. Use abbreviations that are common or well recognized. If you suspect that a certain abbreviation will be misinterpreted by others, do not use it. Keep in mind that should litigation arise from any one of the patients you have previously cared for, you will need clear documentation to support the safety, effectiveness, and excellence of the care that you have provided to all your patients.

A True Story

One busy day in the hematology-oncology clinic, there were two Hispanic female patients with the same last name—Garcia. Their first initials were different—R. vs. H. Both patients were at the clinic for their monthly chemotherapy. The orders for both patients included the drug Cytoxan (cyclophosphamide). The only difference between the two orders was that the dosages were based on the patients' body weight. The nurse was able to avoid a medication error because she diligently asked for the patients' first and last names.

The moral of the story is: Beware of families using a single letter of the alphabet for first names, for example, the Smith family with Alicia, Anna, Alice, Arnold, Anthony, Andy, and so forth. If you use only the last name and a first name initial, all the names will be Smith, A.

▌SOUND-ALIKE OR LOOK-ALIKE DRUGS

The American English language is spoken with distinctive accents, depending on the geographic locale. Also, there are many medical providers educated in non–English-speaking countries whose pronunciation of words is influenced by their accent. To make things worse, there are medications spelled similarly except for two or three letters. The use of abbreviations to describe medications also adds to confusion and potential medication errors. Therefore, be careful how you interpret each written medication order and take additional care when you take medication orders over the telephone.

Recheck each order by asking for the spelling of the medication, or spell the medication as you are taking the order. Also ask for clarification on the dosage form, especially when it involves time-release mechanisms, for example, CR (controlled release), ER (extended release), SR (sustained release) and XL (sustained release). For example, the efficacy of several antihypertensive agents depends on the mechanism by which the therapeutic dose is released.

If you have not written down a record of the care you have provided, it did not happen, or, worse, you did not complete the task!

Be objective with your documentation. Do not document your opinion.

- Keep it legible.
- Keep it brief and accurate.
- Beware of using abbreviations that will only confuse others.
- Draw a single line through any documentation error.
- Do remember to sign your patient's progress notes.
- When in doubt, go through the checks again.

Be careful with abbreviations for the medications; for example, HCTZ = hydrochlorothiazide; CTM = Chlor-Trimeton; INH = isoniazid.

Repeat the order to the source in a question format; for example, Mrs. Angela Dracone is to receive amoxicillin 500 mg t.i.d. for the next 2 weeks?

Double-check the order for dosage form, such as Calan (verapamil) vs. Calan SR (sustained-release verapamil).

TABLE 2–1			
Examples of Medications With Similar-Sounding and Similar-Looking Names			
Triavil	Triphasil	Lodine	Iodine
Zantac	Xanax	Mephyton	Mephenytoin
Cenocort	Senokot	Lanolin	Lanoxin
Alu-Cap	Alupent	DynaCirc	Dynabac
Baclofen	Bactroban	Miconazole	Metronidazole
Atromid	Atrohist	PediaCare	PediaSure
Meclan	Reglan	Phenergan	Phenaphen
Nadolol	Haldol	Phentermine	Phentolamine
Zocor	Psorcon	Xanax	Vanex
Cytoxan	Ciloxan	Zostrix	Zestril
Ophthalgan	Auralgan	BuSpar	Dopar
Ranitidine	Amantadine	Cefotaxime	Cefotetan
Zyrtec	Zantac	Diovan	Dynabac

Table 2–1 lists a few examples of medications that may sound alike and/or look quite similar in writing. No doubt you will find more as your scope of medication administration expands with practical experiences and continuing education.

READING HEALTHCARE PRACTITIONER'S ORDERS

 The use of abbreviations and symbols allows truncation of medication orders.

In the Appendix you will find a table of commonly used abbreviations, their Latin equivalents and English interpretations. These must be remembered for the purpose of interpreting medication orders correctly. Please review extensively.

Prescriptions (Rx) provide the following information:

- Name, signature, address, and license number of the person ordering
- Name of the patient
- Name of the drug
- Unit amount of the drug and its dimensions
- Dose quantity
- Route of administration
- Dosing schedule
- Duration or total quantity of medication
- Number of refills

Here are a few examples of medication orders.

E X A M P L E   1

Order: OxyContin 10 mg 3 tab PO b.i.d.

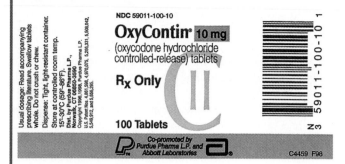

NDC 59011-100-10

OxyContin® 10 mg
(oxycodone hydrochloride
controlled-release) tablets

R$_x$ Only

100 Tablets

Usual dosage: Read accompanying prescribing literature. Swallow tablets whole. Do not crush or chew. Dispense: Tight, light-resistant container. Store at controlled room temp. 15°-30°C (59°-86°F). Dist. by Purdue Pharma L.P., Norwalk, CT 06850-3590 Copyright 1996,1998, Purdue Pharma L.P. U.S. Patent Nos. 4,861,598, 4,970,075, 5,266,331, 5,508,042, 5,549,912, and 5,656,295.

Co-promoted by Purdue Pharma L.P. and Abbott Laboratories

C4459 F98

59011-100-10 1

N3

1. The medication = OxyContin (oxycodone hydrochloride controlled release).
2. The amount of drug = 10.
3. The specific unit or dimension = mg.
4. The dose quantity = 1 tab.
5. The route = PO = by mouth.
6. The dosage schedule = b.i.d. = every 12 hours.

   This order is translated to read: Give to patient 1 tablet of OxyContin 10 mg by mouth every 12 hours.

E X A M P L E   2

Order: Patanol 0.1% 1 drop each eye t.i.d.

1. The medication = Patanol (olopatadine hydrochloride).
2. The amount of drug = 0.1% solution.
3. The specific unit or dimension = drop.
4. The dose quantity = 1 (drop).
5. The route = eye = in lower conjunctival sac.
6. The dosage schedule = t.i.d. = 3 times a day.

   You will give your patient 1 drop of Patanol 0.1% in each eye three times during the day.

E X A M P L E   3

Order: Methergine 0.2 mg IM q2–4hr p.r.n.

1. The medication = Methergine (methylergonovine maleate).
2. The amount of drug = 0.2.
3. The specific unit or dimension = mg.
4. The dose quantity = from dosage calculation.
5. The route = IM = intramuscularly.
6. The dosage schedule = q2–4 hr p.r.n. = every 2–4 hours as needed.

   From this order, your patient will receive an intramuscular injection of Methergine, 0.2 mg every 2 to 4 hours, as needed.

Accuracy in interpretation of a dosage order can be ensured through the use of the five rights.

Orders written on a hospitalized patient's chart consist of almost all components except details concerning provider's address, license number, and refill schedules.

Quite often, the important information supplied on the original package gets covered up with agency labels or other information e.g., what to do if the medication spills on your hand, or how to store the medication.

Apply universal precautions at all times.

Most chemotherapeutic agents are toxic. Wear protective garments to avoid contact with spills, splashes, etc.

Expiration dates are important. Check them and discard the medication if the date has passed.

Lot numbers and bar codes are valuable information if there is a recall on this medication. A USP bar code is typically found on a carton or box containing medication.

READING DRUG LABELS

The US Food and Drug Administration ensures that all licensed drugs are labeled and pertinent information is included. You will find information such as the chemical compound, pharmacodynamics, pharmacokinetics, indications, side and adverse effects, toxicity, and dosages. This information is included within individual packages of each drug. If you take the time to read these drug inserts, practically everything you need to know about the drugs is available.

Frequently, however, these inserts do not accompany the medication to the floor, unit, or agency where you work, so you will need a good reference book on drugs to keep informed about the medications you give to your patients. If you use a unit-dose system where the pharmacy sends medications in small zippered bags, you definitely will not have access to any of the drug package inserts.

Proper storage of medications is essential for maintaining their maximum potency. For example, some of the cephalosporins will break down in as short a time as 4 hours if left unrefrigerated. Another good example is varicella virus, live attenuated (Varivax), the chickenpox vaccine, which must be kept frozen below 0°C. Once reconstituted, Varivax must be discarded after 30 minutes.

You need to know how to extract information from the drug packages (stock or unit dose), so that you will be able to identify and verify that what the pharmacy sends to you is what the healthcare provider ordered. Typically, you will find this information on a drug label:

Trade name (or generic name), chemical name, drug form, dosage (recommended), manufacturer, lot number, storage, expiration date, and important information (Fig. 2–1).

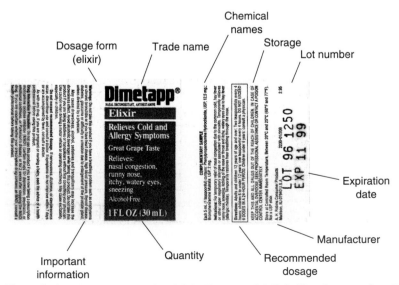

Figure 2–1. *Information on a drug label. (Courtesy of A.H. Robins Company, Inc., Richmond, VA.)*

If you need additional information on any given medication, you can look it up in an up-to-date edition of *Nursing Drug Guides* (NDG), the *Physicians' Desk Reference* (PDR), or an equivalent drug manual. You can always telephone the in-house pharmacist/neighborhood pharmacist or get the information directly from the pharmaceutical company. You can find a listing of pharmaceutical companies' addresses and telephone numbers (some toll free) under the manufacturers' index in most of the drug reference books.

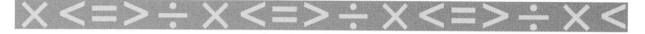

Chapter Summary

This chapter discusses the necessary steps in safe administration of medication dosage. Additionally, it provides guidelines on the process of interpreting medication orders and medication labels. As nursing students, the greatest service you can do for yourself and the patients you care for is to make a habit of diligently learning all you can about any medication that you have never administered. Knowledge serves as the foundation for nurses to provide safe and effective care. Remember that the concept of nursing care is holistic, and that medication administration is only one part of that care.

PROBLEM SET	PROBLEM SET ANSWERS
1. List the three checks.	1. ✔ Before medication is poured ✔ After medication is poured ✔ Before medication is administered
2. List the five rights.	2. Right Patient Right Drug Right Dose Right Route Right Time
3. Discuss the problem with medications that have similar-sounding names.	3. • More reasons to be cautious • More reasons to do the three checks and ensure the five rights

PROBLEM SET	PROBLEM SET ANSWERS

4. Interpret the following medication orders.

4.

a. Auralgan Otic solution 2 drops both ears q2hr p.r.n. pain.

a. Give 2 drops of Auralgan (benzocaine; antipyrine) ear solution, both ears, every 2 hours as needed for pain.

b. Bacitracin oint apply thin layer b.i.d.

b. Apply a thin layer of bacitracin ointment twice a day.

c. Mycelex troches PO 5×/d 5 d.

c. Dissolve Mycelex (clotrimazole) troches in mouth five times a day for 5 days.

d. Estrace vaginal cream apply 1 applicatorful vaginally q.wk.

d. Apply 1 applicatorful of Estrace (estradiol) vaginal cream intravaginally, once a week.

e. Provera 2.5 mg tab PO q.d.

e. Take 1 tablet of Provera (medroxyprogesterone acetate) 2.5 mg by mouth once a day.

Some Facts About Medication Administration

1. The primary role of a nurse is to serve as a patient advocate.
2. Nurses can be sued for nursing malpractice.
3. In addition to the injured patient's suing the nurse in error, doctors involved may also sue the nurse for failure to follow orders.
4. Medication errors make up approximately 30% of all malpractice claims submitted to insurance companies.
5. The leading cause of medication errors is administration of the wrong dosage of medication.
6. The second leading cause of medication error is the administration of a wrong drug to the patient.
7. Another cause of medication error is an omission of a scheduled dose of medication.
8. Administration of IV medication using the wrong rate is yet another leading medication error.
9. Medication administered through a wrong route can potentially be fatal.
10. Administration of medication at the wrong time can potentially harm the patient.
11. Negligence occurs when nurses fail to apply competent nursing practice learned in nursing education programs.
12. Carelessness is a form of negligence.
13. Carelessness in documentation can be construed as careless nursing.
14. Lack of knowledge is a form of negligence.
15. Harm to a patient, based on medication errors, is a major cause of litigation.
16. Failure to follow the established nursing procedures or protocols for dosage administration can lead to litigation.
17. The purpose of a malpractice liability insurance policy, or errors and omission insurance policy, is to protect nurses from financial loss (up to the policy limit) incurred through litigation stemming from patient care issues.
18. Never administer dosage orders that you do not understand.
19. An error in placement of the decimal point can result in compounding errors to dangerous magnitudes, for example,

$$0.001 \quad 0.01 \quad 0.1 \quad 1.0 \quad 10.0 \quad 100.0 \quad 1000.0$$

Moving the decimal point to the right increases the number; moving it to the left decreases it.
20. Placement of a zero to the left of the decimal point clearly defines numbers that are smaller than one, that is,

$$0.135 \quad instead \ of \quad .135$$

Without the zero, the decimal point is diminished and the number threatens to become 135.
21. An intramuscular (IM) or intravenous (IV) injection given improperly can cause serious injury.
22. Medications intended for subcutaneous administration, such as heparin, administered intramuscularly can cause serious injury.
23. When administering medications to your patients, you need to apply the nursing process, which includes assessment, diagnosis, implementation, evaluation, and patient education.
24. Inadequate patient education can lead to litigation.

[3]

> ÷ X < = > ÷ X < = > ÷ X

Understanding Dimensional Analysis

INTRODUCTION

Dimensional Analysis (DA) is *not* a new concept. The concept of manipulating units that describe dimension is heavily used by natural scientists. Currently, the implementation of DA is mostly limited to chemists and scientists in research/experimental laboratories. Dimensional analysis is extremely effective in chemical calculations because most problems in chemistry deploy numerous units of dimensions that range from molecular units through weight units to volumetric units and beyond. Dimensional analysis allows chemists to calculate problems systematically in as few steps as possible for precise and accurate answers.

Dimensional analysis can be equally useful in calculating medication dosages. You do not have to be a chemist to use the concept of DA in your dosage calculations. After all, chemists were once students who learned to use the concept of DA in their chemical calculations. This chapter will provide the basic tools necessary for introducing the concept of DA to solve all dosage calculation problems. Dimensional analysis will be implemented in sample problems to help you follow the concepts.

LEARNING OBJECTIVES

By the end of this chapter, you will be able to:

- Describe what DA is all about

- Incorporate unit equivalencies as conversion factors into dosage problems

- Extract pertinent information from dosage calculation problems

- Utilize pertinent information as extracted conversion factors

- Set up the conversion factors to allow unit cancellation

- Implement unit cancellation in DA

PRETEST: UNIT EQUIVALENCIES	PRETEST ANSWERS

Convert the following measurements to the units indicated.

1. 1 gm to mg (1 gm = 1000 mg)

2. 5 mg to µg (1 mg = 1000 µg)

3. 0.0025 L to ml (1000 ml = 1 L)

4. 10 gr to mg (60 mg = 1 gr)

5. 68 lb to kg (2.2 lb = 1 kg)

6. 15 cc to tsp (5 cc = 1 tsp)

7. 500 cc to L (1000 ml = 1 L), (1 cc = 1 ml)

8. 36.8°C to °F

9. 15 ml to tbsp (5 ml = 1 tsp), (3 tsp = 1 tbsp)

10. 120 µgtt to cc (1 ml = 60 µgtt)

11. 15 ml to gtt (1 ml = 15 gtt)

12. 1 fl oz to ml (1 fl oz = 30 ml)

13. 2 gr to gm (1 gr = 60 mg), (1000 mg = 1 gm)

PRETEST ANSWERS

1. 1000 mg

2. 5000 µg

3. 2.5 ml

4. 600 mg

5. 30.9 kg

6. 3 tsp

7. 0.5 L

8. 98.2°F

9. 1 tbsp

10. 2 cc

11. 225 gtt

12. 30 ml

13. 0.12 gm

PRETEST: UNIT EQUIVALENCIES	PRETEST ANSWERS
14. 25 cc to ml (1 cc = 1 ml)	14. 25 ml
15. 1 tsp to cc (5 cc = 1 tsp)	15. 5 cc
16. 10 km to ft (2.54 cm = 1 inch), (12 inches = 1 ft)	16. 32,808.4 ft
17. 180 lb to kg (2.2 lb = 1 kg)	17. 81.82 kg
18. 500 μg to kg (1,000,000 μg = 1 kg)	18. 0.0005 kg
19. 0.0005 mg to μg (1000 μg = 1 mg)	19. 0.5 μg
20. 98.6°F to Celsius	20. 37°C
21. 25 gr to mg (60 mg = 1 gr)	21. 1500 mg
22. 1 hr to min (60 min = 1 hr)	22. 60 min
23. 20 kg to lb (2.2 lb = 1 kg)	23. 44 lb
24. 1 pt to fl oz (16 fl oz = 1 pt)	24. 16 fl oz
25. 15 gtt to μgtt (1 ml = 15 gtt), (1 ml = 60 μgtt)	25. 60 μgtt
26. 1 pt to ml (1 pt = 16 fl oz), (30 cc = 1 fl oz)	26. 480 ml

You need to be acquainted with unit equivalencies in weight, volume, and distance measurements. You also need to know the unit equivalencies of weights and volumes between metric and nonmetric systems. Other essential unit equivalencies include time and formulas to convert temperature between Celsius and Fahrenheit. Review the unit equivalence tables in the Appendix section.

INFORMATION FROM THE QUESTION AND UNIT EQUIVALENCE TABLES

Typically, the dosage calculation question will provide you with all of the information necessary for solving the problem. From the question, you will be able to extract all of the information necessary for solving the problem. In addition, you are required to use values that represent unit equivalencies between units to carry out the necessary calculations.

- Unit equivalency (U)—the value of equivalencies between two units, for example, 2.2 lb = 1 kg, 5 ml = 1 tsp, 30 ml = 1 fl oz, 1000 μg = 1 mg, 60 min = 1 hr, 15 gtt = 1 ml fluid.

The good news is that there is a built-in pattern within each dosage calculation question. The question will tell you what is ordered for the patient, and then tell you what is available. This chapter will show you how to extract information from the question and solve for desired dimension, that is, what the question is asking you to do.

Depending on the type of question, you will be provided with information pertaining to the order. The following list consists of types of information provided, depending on the dosage scenario:

- Ordered dose—the amount of medication ordered/dose, for example, 1 tab/dose, 2 cap/dose, 500 mg/dose, 5000 U/dose, 100,000 IU/dose.
- Ordered reference dose—the standardized dose of medication based on body weight, body surface area, for example, 10 mg/kg per d, 0.1 mg/kg per min, 20 μg/kg per dose.
- Ordered dosing schedule—the frequency of dosage, for example, q.d. = 1 dose/d, b.i.d. = 2 dose/d, q4hr = every four hours.
- Ordered volume—the volume of medication, usually intravenous medication, for example, 250 ml D_5W (5% dextrose in water), 100 ml NS (normal saline), 1 L lactated Ringer's solution.
- Ordered rate of administration—the delivery rate of medication/time unit, for example, 0.1 ml/min, 20 mg/hr, 5000 U/hr, 1 L/8 hr.
- Ordered duration of time—the length of time required to administer the dosage, for example, give medication over 20 min; give medication for 10 d; give medication for 3 d, then stop 2 d, then repeat another 3 d.

You will always be given an available form of medication in the question, for example, the order is 500 mg, and available is 250 mg/tab.

- Available—available form of medication (PO, SC, IM, IV, etc.), for example, 500 mg/tab, 2 gm/5 ml, 50 mg/250 ml.

Again, depending on the type of dosage calculation question, you will find the following information provided in the question, that is, the same kinds of information you'll find in actual situations.

- Body weight—the patient's body weight, for example, 128 lb, 55.6 kg.
- Body surface area—the patient's body surface area can be obtained from a nomogram (see Appendix) that correlates height, body weight, and body surface area, for example, 1.05 m².
- Intravenous fluids drop factor—the number of drops per ml of fluid, for example, 60 μgtt/ml, 10 gtt/ml, 12 gtt/ml, 15 gtt/ml.

The last part of the question will ask you to calculate something, for example, the number of tabs, the number of tsp, the flow rate (ml/hr). Pay special attention to what the question is asking you to solve, because DA focuses on the desired dimension. For example, How many tab/dose? How many tsp/dose? What is the flow rate in ml/hr?

- Desired dimension—the unit representing the value you are asked to calculate, for example, ml/dose, gtt/dose, ml/hr, gtt/min.

WHAT IS DIMENSIONAL ANALYSIS?

Dimensional analysis is the process of manipulating units, which are descriptions of numbers, in solving mathematical problems. The manipulation process is the cancellation of unwanted units.

 Dimension describes the function of numbers.

What is a unit? A unit is the dimension given to a number. For example, if you are to receive 100, you will immediately ask, 100 what? Depending on your needs, you might want to see a unit such as dollars (to go shopping), points (on the last exam), miles (away from home), years (for peace), hours (of commute), and so forth, thereby adding dimension to the number of 100.

 Unit defines the dimension of numbers.

Medication dosage calculation has little to do with cars and dollars/gallon of gasoline, which are restricted to a mode of transportation. In dosage calculations, we shall be concerned with the units listed in the unit equivalence tables in the Appendix of this book. With DA, you will be shown how correct dosage calculations can be achieved by simple cancellation of all extraneous dimensions (units) in a given problem.

 Medications are measured in weight, volume, and linear units.

 Both metric and US customary systems are used to measure medications (see Appendix).

CONVERSION FACTORS

What is a conversion factor? It is a known unit equivalence. Unit equivalencies are frequently found in unit equivalence tables (Appendix) or derived from the information provided in the question. For example, you know that 1 gr equals 60 to 65 mg. To keep things simple, we shall use 60 mg to equal 1 gr. The conversion factor for this unit equivalence can be written as:

 Conversion factors are unit equivalencies written in a fraction format.

$$\frac{60 \text{ mg}}{1 \text{ gr}} \quad \text{or} \quad \frac{1 \text{ gr}}{60 \text{ mg}}$$

 There are two sources of information for derivation of conversion factors:
1. Unit equivalence tables
2. Information provided in dosage problems

It may clarify matters for you to conceptualize the above conversion factor fractions as 60 mg per grain, and vice versa. We have not introduced any value changes to the unit. Instead, we simply rewrote the unit equivalence of 60 mg = 1 gr in a fraction format.

Similarly, all unit equivalencies can be rewritten as conversion factors. Additionally, conversion factors may be derived from information provided in a given question. For example, the Tylenol dosage of "Tylenol 160 mg/5 ml"

 Extracted conversion factors are conversion factors derived from information provided in the dosage problem.

Read and interpret questions carefully.

from a dosage problem can be written in two formats of conversion factors:

$$\frac{160 \text{ mg}}{5 \text{ ml}} \quad \text{or} \quad \frac{5 \text{ ml}}{160 \text{ mg}}$$

Essentially, the conversion factor is extracted from information provided in the dosage problem. Therefore, the term "extracted conversion factor" will be used in the examples to delineate them from the ones derived from unit equivalence tables.

Here are some examples to demonstrate the process:

E X A M P L E   1

1000 ml = 1 qt

Conversion factor: $\dfrac{1000 \text{ ml}}{1 \text{ qt}}$ or $\dfrac{1 \text{ qt}}{1000 \text{ ml}}$

E X A M P L E   2

15 gtt = 1 ml

Conversion factor: $\dfrac{15 \text{ gtt}}{1 \text{ ml}}$ or $\dfrac{1 \text{ ml}}{15 \text{ gtt}}$

E X A M P L E   3

2.2 lb = 1 kg

Conversion factor: $\dfrac{2.2 \text{ lb}}{1 \text{ kg}}$ or $\dfrac{1 \text{ kg}}{2.2 \text{ lb}}$

E X A M P L E   4

1 mg = 1000 μg

Conversion factor: $\dfrac{1 \text{ mg}}{1000 \text{ }\mu g}$ or $\dfrac{1000 \text{ }\mu g}{1 \text{ mg}}$

You will notice that there are two different conversion factors derived from the same unit equivalence.

M I N I   Q U I Z

Which conversion factor is applicable in dosage calculation?

Answer: Choose the one that allows you to cancel unwanted units.

DIMENSIONAL ANALYSIS UNIT CANCELLATION: UNIT EQUIVALENCE CONVERSION FACTOR

In the Pretest, the questions ask you to convert one type of unit to another. We shall demonstrate how you can use DA to carry out unit conversions.

You can follow these steps to convert one unit to another with unit equivalence (equiv):

1. Identify the desired unit dimension or units.
2. Keep the desired unit dimension in proper numerator (and denominator) orientation.
3. Identify the link or unit equivalence(s).
4. Identify the unwanted dimension or units.
5. Cancel unwanted units.
6. Perform the arithmetic.

Always write the dimension(s) that you are seeking (the desired dimension or the answer) in the proper numerator/denominator orientation, that is, N/D in proper orientation.

Here are a few examples to demonstrate the DA process:

E X A M P L E   1

How many mg are there in 5 kg?
What is the link between mg and kg?
The link is the unit equivalence: 1 kg = 1000 mg.

Format:	A	B
Rewritten as conversion factor:	$\dfrac{1 \text{ kg}}{1000 \text{ mg}}$ or	$\dfrac{1000 \text{ mg}}{1 \text{ kg}}$

Desired unit dimension in the answer: mg

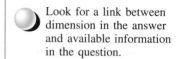
Look for a link between dimension in the answer and available information in the question.

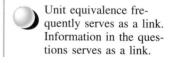
Unit equivalence frequently serves as a link. Information in the questions serves as a link.

Therefore, you must keep the dimension mg as the numerator. Which conversion factor, A or B, will allow you to cancel kg to have mg as the end result? The only one that allows mg to remain as the numerator is the conversion factor B.

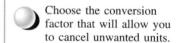
Choose the conversion factor that will allow you to cancel unwanted units.

CORRECT setup: Allows cancellation of unwanted unit, kg.

$$\frac{1000 \text{ mg}}{1 \text{ kg}} \times 5 \text{ kg} = 5000 \text{ mg}$$

$\underset{\text{with desired unit}}{\text{Unit equiv (U)}} \times \underset{\text{unit (A)}}{\text{Available}} = \text{Answer}$

The dimension, kg, is canceled.

If you did not properly orient your conversion factor, your answer might have looked like this:

$$\frac{1 \text{ kg}}{1000 \text{ mg}} \times 5 \text{ kg} = \frac{5 \text{ kg}^2}{1000 \text{ mg}} = \frac{\text{kg}^2}{200 \text{ mg}} \quad \text{[Try again!]}$$

None of the units can be canceled.

E X A M P L E   2

Convert 100 lb to kg.
   Unit equivalence: 2.2 lb = 1 kg is the link between lb and kg.

Format:	A	B
Conversion factors:	$\dfrac{2.2 \text{ lb}}{1 \text{ kg}}$ or	$\dfrac{1 \text{ kg}}{2.2 \text{ lb}}$

Desired unit: kg

$$D \times U \times U \times A = Ans$$

$$A \times U \times U \times D = Ans$$

The correct conversion factors are:

$$\frac{60\ sec}{min} \quad or \quad \frac{min}{60\ sec}$$

$$\frac{60\ min}{hr} \quad or \quad \frac{hr}{60\ min}$$

$$\frac{24\ hr}{d} \quad or \quad \frac{d}{24\ hr}$$

$$\frac{7\ d}{wk} \quad or \quad \frac{wk}{7\ d}$$

① $$\frac{60\ sec}{1\ min} \times \frac{24\ hr}{1\ d} \times \frac{7\ d}{1\ wk}$$

$$\times \frac{60\ min}{1\ hr} \times 1\ wk$$

② $$\frac{24\ hr}{1\ d} \times \frac{7\ d}{1\ wk} \times \frac{60\ min}{1\ hr}$$

$$\times \frac{60\ sec}{1\ min} \times 1\ wk$$

$$A \times U \times U \times D = Ans$$

CORRECT setup: Keeping c as the numerator.

$$\frac{1\ c}{8\ \cancel{fl\ oz}} \times \frac{1\ \cancel{fl\ oz}}{30\ \cancel{cc}} \times \frac{1000\ \cancel{cc}}{1\ \cancel{L}} \times 1\ \cancel{L} = 4.17\ c$$

or, in any order that allows unwanted units to cancel, for example,

$$1\ \cancel{L} \times \frac{1000\ \cancel{cc}}{1\ \cancel{L}} \times \frac{1\ \cancel{fl\ oz}}{30\ \cancel{cc}} \times \frac{1\ c}{8\ \cancel{fl\ oz}} = 4.17\ c$$

E X A M P L E   7

How many sec are there in a wk? There are four links between sec and wk:

Unit equivalencies: 60 sec = 1 min
60 min = 1 hr
24 hr = 1 d
7 d = 1 wk

Write all the conversion factors for these unit equivalencies.

or

or

or

or

Desired unit: sec

CORRECT setup: Allows cancellation of wk, d, hr, and min, leaving sec as the end result.

$$1\ \cancel{wk} \times \frac{7\ \cancel{d}}{1\ \cancel{wk}} \times \frac{24\ \cancel{hr}}{1\ \cancel{d}} \times \frac{60\ \cancel{min}}{1\ \cancel{hr}} \times \frac{60\ sec}{1\ \cancel{min}} = 604,800\ sec$$

$$A \quad \times \quad U \quad \times \quad U \quad \times \quad U \quad \times \quad D \quad = \quad Ans$$

For practice, rewrite the above string of conversion factors in two different arrangements.

1. _____

2. _____

Let's look at this example again. If you know that there are 3600 sec in an hr, you can certainly eliminate a link (step) in the setup:

$$1\ \cancel{wk} \times \frac{7\ \cancel{d}}{1\ \cancel{wk}} \times \frac{24\ \cancel{hr}}{1\ \cancel{d}} \times \frac{3600\ \cancel{sec}}{1\ \cancel{hr}} = 604,800\ sec$$

The end result is the same. Of course, if you are a collector of trivial information, you may know that there are 604,800 sec in a week.

EX

Orde
Avai
Calcula
Infor

25 mg/
50 mg/
10 ml/

Desi

CORRE

$\dfrac{1\ r}{50\ }$
Avail

EX

Orde
Avai
Calcula

M I
What is

Put a c
provide

250 mg
500 mg
4 doses
10 d

Extr

Desi
CORRE

$\dfrac{1\ ta}{500}$
Avail

MINI QUIZ

Could you solve this problem with even fewer conversion factors?

Answer: yes

DIMENSIONAL ANALYSIS UNIT CANCELLATION: EXTRACTED CONVERSION FACTORS

The focus of this section is to use examples of dosage calculation questions to demonstrate the process of:

- Analyzing dosage calculation questions
- Developing a list of information provided in the question
- Selecting the pertinent facts from the information provided
- Utilizing the pertinent information as extracted conversion factors
- Incorporating both the derived unit equivalence and the extracted conversion factors
- Conducting DA to cancel unwanted units

Akin to mathematical problems, medication dosage calculation problems will provide you with all the information necessary for solving the problems—with the exception of unit equivalencies. Frequently, however, dosage problems provide information far beyond what you need to solve them. The additional information serves to add realism to the problem; however, it also tends to confuse and tax your analytical abilities. Therefore, it is extremely important that you read the problem carefully, analyzing the available information and selecting the data pertinent to solving the problem.

We recommend that you systematically analyze each dosage calculation problem by posing the following questions:

- What is the problem asking me to do?
- What information does the problem give me?
- Which portion of the information do I really need?
- What other information, for example, unit equivalencies, do I need to solve this question?

Here are examples of dosage calculation problems that furnish all necessary information about the dosage ordered and the dosage available. Problems such as these follow two basic patterns:

$$\textbf{Ordered (Desired)} \times \textbf{Available (Have)} = \textbf{Answer (Ans)}$$
$$O \qquad \times \qquad A \qquad = \qquad Ans$$

or,

$$\textbf{Available (Have)} \times \textbf{Ordered (Desired)} = \textbf{Answer (Ans)}$$
$$A \qquad \times \qquad O \qquad = \qquad Ans$$

Select the pertinent facts from the information in the dosage problems.

Dosage problems are composed of two parts. The first part states the medication as ordered, and the second part notes what is available for you to complete the order.

Do not lose sight of what the dosage problem is asking you to solve.

EXAMPLE 7

Ordered: Lidocaine 2 gm IV in 500 ml of D_5W

Available: Lidocaine 20 mg/ml in 50 ml single-use vial

Calculate the number of vials you would need for this solution.

Put a check mark in the box next to the pertinent piece(s) of information provided.

2 gm/dose	(Ordered)	☐
2 gm/500 ml	(Ordered)	☐
20 mg/ml	(Available)	☐
50 ml/vial	(Available)	☐

Extracted conversion factors: $\dfrac{50\ ml}{vial}$; $\dfrac{20\ mg}{ml}$; $\dfrac{2\ gm}{dose}$

Unit equivalence conversion factor: $\dfrac{1\ gm}{1000\ mg}$

Desired unit: vial

CORRECT setup:

$$\frac{1\ vial}{50\ \cancel{ml}} \times \frac{1\ \cancel{ml}}{20\ \cancel{mg}} \times \frac{1000\ \cancel{mg}}{1\ \cancel{gm}} \times \frac{2\ \cancel{gm}}{dose} = 2\ vials$$

Available × Available × Unit equiv conversion factor × Ordered = Answer

The next example demonstrates a more difficult problem. Again, do not dwell on the dosage administration topic of intravenous drip rates, which is unfamiliar to beginning nursing students. Remember that the focus is on the extraction of information, the development of the conversion factor, and the unit of cancellation.

EXAMPLE 8

Ordered: Lidocaine 1 mg/min IV

Available: Lidocaine 2 gm/500ml D_5W

Calculate the flow rate (ml/hr) for this patient using a microdrip chamber set that delivers 60 microdrops/ml (60 µgtt/ml).

Put a check mark in the box next to the pertinent piece(s) of information.

1 mg/min	(Ordered)	☐
2 gm/500 ml	(Available)	☐
60 µgtt/ml	(Unit equivalence)	☐

Extracted conversion factors: $\dfrac{1\ mg}{1\ min}$; $\dfrac{2\ gm}{500\ ml}$

Unit equivalence conversion factors: $\dfrac{1\ gm}{1000\ mg}$; $\dfrac{60\ min}{hr}$

Desired unit: $\dfrac{ml}{hr}$ (as numerator) (as denominator)

(Left sidebar)

Answers:

 ☑

☐ Extraneous

☑

☑

There are two different unit dimensions in this problem, that is; mg and gm. You can use either of the two unit equivalencies: 1000 mg = 1 gm or 1 gm = 0.001 mg.

$A \times A \times U \times O = Ans$

You can solve any dosage calculation problem, even if you do not know how to administer the drug as ordered.

Answers:

 ☑

 ☑

☐ Extraneous

Keep the fraction format of desired unit dimensions in the same numerator to denominator orientation, that is,

$$\frac{Numerator}{Denominator} = \frac{ml}{hr}$$

and place it first in your setup.

CORRECT setup:

$$\frac{500\ \text{ml}}{2\ \cancel{\text{gm}}} \times \frac{1\ \cancel{\text{gm}}}{1000\ \cancel{\text{mg}}} \times \frac{1\ \cancel{\text{mg}}}{1\ \cancel{\text{min}}} \times \frac{60\ \cancel{\text{min}}}{\text{hr}} = 15\ \text{ml/hr}$$

$$A \times U \times O \times U = Ans$$

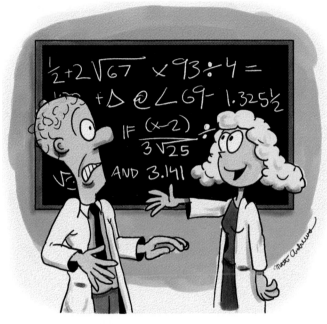

"I'M GLAD WE'VE BEEN ABLE TO SIMPLIFY THE FORMULA!"

The examples you have examined demonstrate that all medication dosage problems can be solved using DA to set up conversion factors (extracted or unit equivalence). Extracted conversion factors can be categorized as ordered and available. Most dosage problems can be solved by applying either of the following setups:

Available × Ordered = Answer

or,

Available × Ordered × Unit equiv conversion factor = Answer

No amount of mastery of DA can correct mathematical errors.

Chapter Summary

The concept of dimensional analysis has been introduced with sample problems to implement the concept. Simply put, DA is a process of manipulating units. This process involves cancellation of units in conversion factors. The role of the problem solver is to derive conversion factors from unit equivalency tables and/or information from the questions.

It is difficult to learn anything new. You may have already noticed that you can adopt DA in small, independent steps. For example, you can set up the pertinent information provided by the question for unit conversion (that is, O × U = partial answer), and then carry the answer to the next step (that is, partial answer × A = Ans).

Also, if you are learning DA for the first time, it may make dosage calculations easier, enabling you to solve at least a small part of each dosage problem by this method. In time, you will be able to correctly set up cancellation in a single step. As you gain experience in implementing DA, beware of the urge to set up the problems without writing down the respective units next to the numbers. To avoid errors, always write the units next to the numbers. Make sure you are multiplying and dividing a correct set of numerators and denominators. The only fail-safe method is to make sure that all the unwanted units cancel. Otherwise, you may get an answer that is quite *wrong*.

Beginning users of DA are frequently plagued by the following problems:

Problem. The orientation of conversion units.
Solution. Always put the desired unit at the beginning of your setup. Remember to orient the desired unit dimension(s) in the proper numerator to denominator orientation.

Problem. All unwanted units cannot be canceled.
Solution. Be sure to include the necessary conversion factors for unit equivalence conversion in your setup. Remember to orient the conversion factors (extractions or unit equivalencies) in the proper numerator and denominator orientation to allow the units to cancel.

If you are having difficulty with the information provided in this chapter, review the examples carefully! Here is a summary of the process of DA.

1. Read the question carefully.
2. Select the pertinent data from the information provided in the problem.
3. Determine the desired end result dimension, that is, the unit wanted in the answer.
4. Develop the necessary conversion factors from the unit equivalencies and/or information provided in the problem.
5. Make sure the desired unit dimension remains as a numerator, that is, on the top of the fraction (or numerator/denominator).
6. Set up the conversion factors to cancel the unwanted units in each conversion factor.
7. Cancel all the unwanted units.
8. Carry out the necessary mathematical calculations.
9. Always double-check your work.

PROBLEM SET

Solve the following unit equivalency problems.

1. How many cc in ½ tsp?

2. Convert 20 gtt to cc (15 gtt = 1 cc).

3. How many qt in 4 fl oz?

4. Convert 1.5 inches to cm.

PROBLEM SET ANSWERS

1. 2.5 cc

2. 1.3 cc

3. 0.125 qt

4. 3.81 cm

PROBLEM SET	PROBLEM SET ANSWERS

5. Convert 0.05 gm to μg.

5. 50,000 μg

6. Convert 0.0025 L to cc.

6. 2.5 cc

7. Convert 0.25 gm to gr.

7. 4.17 gr

8. Convert ¹⁄₄₀ gr to mg.

8. 1.5 mg

9. How many tsp in 2 tbsp?

9. 6 tsp

10. Convert 88 lb to kg.

10. 40 kg

Solve these problems by making sure you list all the available information provided; extract the conversion factors from the information provided; and set up the conversion factors for the cancellation of the unwanted units.

1. Ordered: Furosemide 40 mg PO.
   Available: Furosemide 20 mg tablets

   Calculate the number of tablets per dose.

1. 40 mg/dose; 20 mg/tab;
   $\dfrac{40 \text{ mg}}{\text{dose}}; \dfrac{20 \text{ mg}}{\text{tab}}$

   2 tab/dose

2. Ordered: Tylenol 500 mg PO stat.
   Available: Tylenol (acetaminophen) 500 mg tablets

   Calculate the number of tablets per dose.

2. 500 mg/dose;
   500 mg/tab;
   $\dfrac{500 \text{ mg}}{\text{dose}}; \dfrac{500 \text{ mg}}{\text{tab}}$

   1 tab/dose

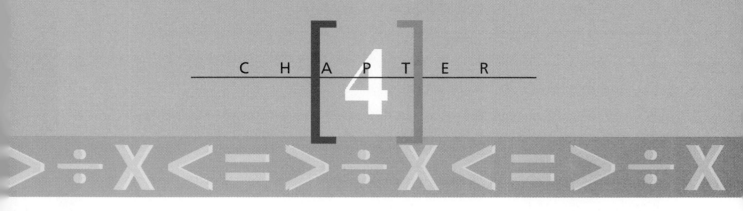

Fundamental Use of Dimensional Analysis

INTRODUCTION

In Chapter 3, the concept of dimensional analysis (DA) was introduced. With DA, you can solve dosage calculation problems by setting up a series of conversion factors. The process of unit cancellation in removing unwanted units in conversion factors was demonstrated. Finally, Chapter 3 showed that dosage problems can be solved in a single step by carrying out necessary multiplication and division of remaining numbers and units. In this chapter, DA will be used in solving dosage problems related to oral, rectal, and topical, as well as eye and ear medications, which are usually the first medications a nursing student administers.

The process that involves extracting pertinent information from questions, deriving conversion factors, and cancelling units will be employed in solving medication dosage problems. Realistic scenarios of indications, dosage, and administration will be provided for all of the dosage calculation examples.

Additionally, the concept of percent (%) concentration is discussed to provide you with a basis for solving dosage problems of medications that require this kind of measurement.

(Continued)

LEARNING OBJECTIVES

By the end of this chapter, you will be able to apply DA to calculate dosages for:

- Oral medications, including tablets, geltabs, capsules, reconstituted powders, liquids, swish and swallows, and inhalers

- Topical medications, including gels, lotions, ointments, pastes, and patches

- Ear and eye drops

- Medications for rectal and vaginal administration, including suppositories, enemas, and irrigations

Some Facts About Medication Dosage Calculation Using DA

1. The desired unit dimension is what the dosage problem is asking you to find.
2. Conversion factors can be arranged in two distinctly different formats.
3. Unit equivalencies are commonly used as conversion factors.
4. Information provided in the dosage problem can be used to determine conversion factors.
5. Information provided in dosage problems can be categorized as either ordered or available dosages.
6. In the setup to cancel unwanted units, the desired unit dimension (unit) must be kept as the numerator.
7. Most dosage problems can be solved by using the pertinent conversion factors:

$$\text{Available} \times \text{Ordered} = \text{Answer}$$

8. Frequently, unit equivalence conversion factors are used:

$$\text{Available} \times \text{Ordered} \times \text{Unit equiv conversion factor} = \text{Answer}$$

9. A good way of extracting the pertinent information from a problem is to look for the desired unit dimension(s).
10. The five rights and the three checks are crucial safety measures that help to prevent medication errors.
11. It is a prudent safety measure to look up medications that are unfamiliar to you.
12. The abbreviation for oral route is PO.
13. The abbreviation for dosing three times a day is t.i.d.
14. The abbreviation for bedtime is h.s.
15. The abbreviation for every hour is q.h.
16. The abbreviation for left eye is O.S.
17. Always round calculated answers to the nearest measurable unit.
18. Long-acting, extended-release, or timed-release oral medications cannot be cut or crushed.
19. It is easier to measure volume in ml than tsp (for example, 1 to 4 ml versus ¼, ½, ¾ tsp).

If you are having any problems with the Pretest, you will need to review Chapter 3, as well as the unit equivalencies and the Latin-English abbreviation tables in the Appendix. The following checklist will guide you through most of the problems in this chapter:

✔ Interpret the problem appropriately, that is, determine what you are solving for.

✔ Extract pertinent facts and use them as conversion factors.

✔ Apply unit equivalence conversion factors as needed.

✔ Remember that most problems can be solved by using the pertinent conversion factor(s):

$$\textbf{Ordered} \times \textbf{Available} = \textbf{Answer}$$
$$O \quad \times \quad A \quad = \quad Ans$$

or

$$\textbf{Ordered} \times \textbf{Available} \times \textbf{Univ equiv} = \textbf{Answer}$$
$$O(s) \quad \times \quad A(s) \quad \times \quad U(s) \quad = \quad Ans$$

CALCULATIONS FOR ADMINISTRATION OF ORAL MEDICATIONS

Dosage Form	Definition
Tablets, Caplets, Geltabs, Gelcaps, Filmtabs	Compressed mixtures of medication plus extender, delivered in powdered, liquid, or crystalline forms, with a protective covering around the medication that allows ease of swallowing.
Capsules	Encapsulated medications (powder or liquid) with two overlapping half-shells for enclosure.
Powders	Crystalline forms of medication. The powdered form of a medication is seldom given orally because it may cause choking. Most powdered medications need to be reconstituted to a liquid or solution form for administration (see Chapters 5 and 6), except in topical applications, for example, fungal foot powder.
Liquids, including suspensions, syrups, elixirs, swish and swallows	Powdered medications are dissolved or suspended in a diluent, such as water. Additional ingredients, for example, glucose, flavoring, and food coloring compounds, may be added to improve palatability, visual appeal, odor, efficacy, shelf-life, stability, and general marketability.
Inhalers and sprays	Liquid forms of medication contained in dispensers specially designed to deliver a calibrated dose of medication with each depression or pumping action.

Tablets, Geltabs, Caplets, and Capsules

The following examples demonstrate the use of DA to solve common dosage calculation problems in oral medication administration.

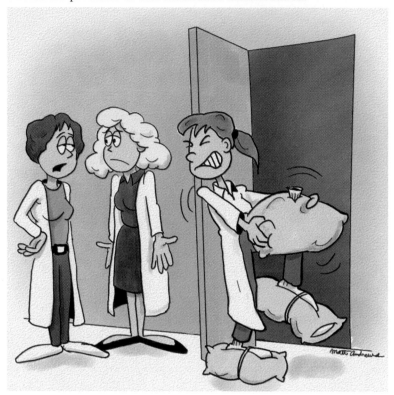

"WHENEVER JUDY BRINGS MR. THOMPSON
HIS NITROGLYCERIN, SHE TAKES THESE
PRECAUTIONS.... I WONDER HOW SHE PASSED
HER PHARMACOLOGY COURSE!"

EXAMPLE 1

Ordered: Vanex Forte 1 tab PO b.i.d. p.r.n.

Available: Vanex Forte (phenylpropanolamine HCl; phenylephrine HCl; chlorpheniramine maleate; pyrilamine maleate) tab

NDC 12463-125-01

Vanex® Forte

LONG-ACTING ANTIHISTAMINE
DECONGESTANT CAPLETS

Each caplet contains:

Phenylpropanolamine HCl	50 mg
Phenylephrine HCl	10 mg
Pyrilamine Maleate	25 mg
Chlorpheniramine Maleate	4 mg

100 CAPLETS

Abana

Manufactured For:
ABANA PHARMACEUTICALS, INC.
BIRMINGHAM, AL 35209

Manufactured By:
ANABOLIC, INC.
IRVINE, CA 92714

CAUTION: Federal law prohibits dispensing without prescription.

DOSAGE: ADULTS 1 caplet 2-3 times daily. CHILDREN (6-12y) 1/2 caplet 2-3 times daily. CHILDREN (under 6y) only as directed by physician. Do not crush or chew caplets. Do not exceed recommended daily dosage. For complete prescribing information see accompanying insert.

Store at controlled room temperature 59°-86°F (15°-30°C). Protect from light.

6277-01A

EXP

LOT

3   12463 12501   6

Calculate the number of tab/dose.

   Pertinent information available: 1 tab/dose.
   Unit equivalency conversion: None needed
   Desired unit: tab/dose

CORRECT setup: None needed

   Answer: 1 tab/dose

Some medications are available in single-strength dosage forms, and they are ordered with a designated dosage. This is an example of one.

EXAMPLE 2

   Ordered: BuSpar 10 mg PO t.i.d.
   Available: BuSpar (buspirone HCl) 5-mg tab

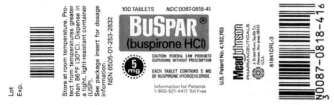

Calculate the number of tab/dose.

   Pertinent information provided: 10 mg/dose; 5 mg/tab
   Unit equivalency conversion: None needed
   Desired unit: tab/dose

CORRECT setup:

$$\frac{\text{tab}}{5 \text{ mg}} \times \frac{10 \text{ mg}}{\text{dose}} = 2 \text{ tab/dose}$$

As long as the unwanted units cancel, the position of the conversion factor in the setup does not alter the outcome.

A × O = Ans

EXAMPLE 3

   Ordered: Fosamax 40 mg PO q.d for 6 mo
   Available: Alendronate 40-mg tab
Calculate the number of tab/dose.

   Pertinent information provided: 40 mg/dose; 40 mg/tab
   Unit equivalency conversion: None needed
   Desired unit: tab/dose

CORRECT setup:

$$\frac{\text{tab}}{40 \text{ mg}} \times \frac{40 \text{ mg}}{\text{dose}} = 1 \text{ tab/dose}$$

Often, medications are ordered by their trade name, but they are available only by their generic name. Check a drug book for the correct medication names.

A × O = Ans

EXAMPLE 4

   Ordered: BuSpar 15 mg 1 tab PO q.h.s. for 2 wk then b.i.d.
   Available: Buspirone HCl 10-mg tab

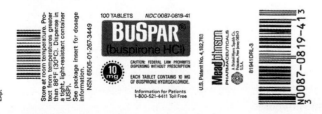

BuSpar is the trade name for buspirone HCl.

Calculate the number of tab/dose.
   Pertinent information provided: 15 mg/dose; 10 mg/tab
   Unit equivalency conversion: None needed
   Desired Unit: tab/dose

CORRECT setup:

 A × O = Ans

$$\frac{\text{tab}}{10 \ \cancel{\text{mg}}} \times \frac{15 \ \cancel{\text{mg}}}{\text{dose}} = 1\frac{1}{2} \ \text{tab/dose}$$

E X A M P L E   5

   Ordered: Procardia XL 60 mg PO q.d.
   Available: Procardia XL (extended-release nifedipine) 30-mg tab
Calculate the number of tab/dose.
   Pertinent information provided: 30 mg/tab; 60 mg/dose
   Unit equivalency conversion: None needed
   Desired unit: tab/dose

 Cutting or crushing medication, such as Procardia XL, destroys the sustained-release or extended-release mechanism.

 A × O = Ans

CORRECT setup:

$$\frac{\text{tab}}{30 \ \cancel{\text{mg}}} \times \frac{60 \ \cancel{\text{mg}}}{\text{dose}} = 2 \ \text{tab/dose}$$

E X A M P L E   6

   Ordered: Colchicine 0.01 gr PO q.d. for 14 d
   Available: Colchicine 0.6-mg tab
Calculate the number of tab/dose.
   Pertinent information provided. 0.01 gr/dose; 0.6 mg/tab
   Unit equivalency conversion: 60 mg/gr
   Desired unit: tab/dose

 To convert gr of colchicine to mg, extract the unit equivalence conversion factor, that is, 60 to 65 mg/gr.

 A × U × O = Ans

CORRECT setup:

$$\frac{\text{tab}}{0.6 \ \cancel{\text{mg}}} \times \frac{60 \ \cancel{\text{mg}}}{1 \ \cancel{\text{gr}}} \times \frac{0.01 \ \cancel{\text{gr}}}{\text{dose}} = 1 \ \text{tab/dose}$$

E X A M P L E   7

   Ordered: Tylenol 500 mg 2 gelcap PO q.i.d.
   Available: Tylenol (acetaminophen) 500-mg gelcap
Calculate the number of gm/dose.

M I N I   Q U I Z

What is the problem asking you to do?

Answer: To convert Tylenol dosage from mg/dose to gm/dose.

 Convert mg to gm by using the unit equivalence.

   Pertinent information provided: 500 mg/cap; 2 cap/dose
   Unit equivalence: 1 gm/1000 mg
   Desired unit: gm/dose

CORRECT setup:

$$\frac{500 \text{ mg}}{\text{cap}} \times \frac{2 \text{ cap}}{\text{dose}} \times \frac{1 \text{ gm}}{1000 \text{ mg}} = 1 \text{ gm/dose}$$

    A × O × U = Ans

or,

$$\frac{500 \text{ mg}}{\text{cap}} \times \frac{2 \text{ cap}}{\text{dose}} \times \frac{0.001 \text{ gm}}{1 \text{ mg}} = 1 \text{ gm/dose}$$

    A × O × U = Ans

E X A M P L E   8

Ordered: Flagyl 500 mg 4 tab PO single dose
Available: Flagyl (metronidazole) 500-mg tab
Calculate the gm of Flagyl per dose.
  Pertinent information provided: 500 mg/tab; 4 tab/dose
  Unit equivalency conversion: 1000 mg/gm
  Desired unit: gm/dose

CORRECT setup:

$$\frac{500 \text{ mg}}{\text{tab}} \times \frac{4 \text{ tab}}{\text{dose}} \times \frac{1 \text{ gm}}{1000 \text{ mg}} = 2 \text{ gm/dose}$$

    A × O × U = Ans

E X A M P L E   9

Ordered: Amoxicillin 250 mg PO q.i.d. for 10 d
Available: Amoxicillin 250-mg capsule
Calculate the number of gm of amoxicillin needed for 10 d.

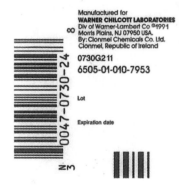

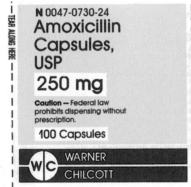

N 0047-0730-24
Amoxicillin Capsules, USP
250 mg
Caution — Federal law prohibits dispensing without prescription.
100 Capsules
 WARNER CHILCOTT

Each capsule contains amoxicillin trihydrate equivalent to 250 mg amoxicillin.
Usual Adult Dosage— 250 or 500 mg every 8 hours. See package insert.
PHARMACY STOCK PACKAGE
Dispense in a tight, light-resistant container as defined in the USP.
Store below 30°C (86°F). Protect from moisture.
0730J030

M I N I   Q U I Z
What is the problem asking you to calculate?

  Pertinent information provided: 250 mg/dose; 4 dose/d; 10 d
  Unit equivalency conversion: 1 gm/1000 mg
  Desired unit: gm

CORRECT setup:

$$\frac{250 \text{ mg}}{\text{dose}} \times \frac{1 \text{ gm}}{1000 \text{ mg}} \times \frac{4 \text{ dose}}{\text{d}} \times 10 \text{ d} = 10 \text{ gm}$$

Answer: The total amount of medication needed over the 10 d, in gm.

 Read and interpret each problem carefully.

 O × U × Os × Ot = Ans (Os is the ordered dosing schedule, Ot is the ordered length of time.)

Liquids, Suspensions, Syrups, Elixirs, Swish and Swallows, and Reconstituted Powders

The physical flowing nature of liquids makes them fluid. Therefore, liquid medications are measured in volume, by using the metric and nonmetric systems. You are advised to review the Appendix for unit equivalencies between metric and nonmetric volume measurements.

What is the difference between cc and ml in volume measurements? The unit cc (cubic centimeter) accounts for mass and density in measuring volume, that is, mass = volume × density. The unit ml (milliliter) is a direct measurement of volume. Because the density of water is 1 at standard temperature and pressure, cc = ml. The two units, cc and ml, are used interchangeably in dosage calculations involving volume measurements.

In the following examples, DA will be implemented to demonstrate dosage calculation of liquid oral medications.

 Shake the suspension prior to administration. If the suspension is not shaken, the amount of medication in the dose administered will not be correct. The medication will be "suspended" in the diluent, and gravity will make the medication settle to the bottom of the bottle.

E X A M P L E   1

Ordered: Diphenhydramine 25 mg PO q.i.d. p.r.n.
Available: Hydramine Elixir 12.5 mg/tsp suspension

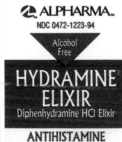

Calculate the amount in ml/dose.
    Pertinent information provided: 25 mg/dose; 12.5 mg/tsp
    Unit equivalency conversion: 5 ml/tsp
    Desired unit: ml/dose

CORRECT setup:

 U × A × O = Ans

$$\frac{5\ \text{ml}}{\text{tsp}} \times \frac{\text{tsp}}{12.5\ \text{mg}} \times \frac{25\ \text{mg}}{\text{dose}} = 10\ \text{ml/dose}$$

Syrup frequently contains a nutritive sweetener, such as fructose or sucrose. Patients who have diabetes may need sugar-free formulations.

EXAMPLE 2

Ordered: Symmetrel 50 mg PO b.i.d.
Available: Amantadine HCl 50 mg/tsp syrup

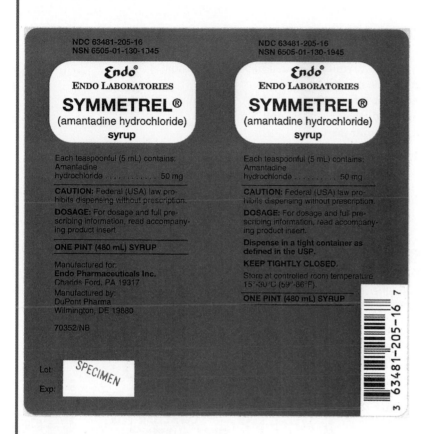

Calculate the number of tsp/dose
   Pertinent information provided: 50 mg/dose; 50 mg/tsp
   Unit equivalency conversion: None needed
   Desired unit: tsp/dose

CORRECT setup:

$$\frac{\text{tsp}}{50 \text{ mg}} \times \frac{50 \text{ mg}}{\text{dose}} = 1 \text{ tsp/dose}$$

A × O = Ans

EXAMPLE 3

Ordered: Nizoral 50 mg PO b.i.d.
Available: Ketoconazole 200 mg/tsp compounded by the pharmacist from tab to suspension
Calculate the number of ml/dose.
   Pertinent information provided: 50 mg/dose; 200 mg/tsp
   Unit equivalency conversion: 5 ml/tsp.
   Desired unit: ml/dose

Compounding is a process used by pharmacists to convert medication from one form to another, for example, tablet to liquid, powder to solution or suspension.

$$U \times A \times O = Ans$$

CORRECT setup:

$$\frac{5 \text{ ml}}{\text{tsp}} \times \frac{\text{tsp}}{200 \text{ mg}} \times \frac{50 \text{ mg}}{\text{dose}} = 1.25 \text{ ml/dose}$$

E X A M P L E   4

Ordered: Erythromycin 250 mg PO q.i.d.
Available: Erythromycin 200 mg/tsp suspension
Calculate the number of ml/dose.
    Pertinent information provided: 250 mg/dose; 200 mg/tsp
    Unit equivalency conversion: 5 ml/tsp
    Desired unit: ml/dose

Try placing the conversion factors in an order other than the one presented, for example, O × U × A.

CORRECT setup:

$$\frac{\text{tsp}}{200 \text{ mg}} \times \frac{5 \text{ ml}}{1 \text{ tsp}} \times \frac{250 \text{ mg}}{\text{dose}} = 6.25 \text{ ml/dose}$$

$$A \times U \times O = Ans$$

E X A M P L E   5

Ordered: Ceclor* 250 mg PO t.i.d.
Available: Cefaclor 125 mg/tsp suspension

Cancel and/or reduce the fractions to make them easier to multiply.

NDC 0002-5057-68
150 mL (When Mixed)   **M-5057**

℞   *Lilly*

CECLOR®
CEFACLOR FOR
ORAL SUSPENSION, USP
125 mg
per 5 mL

CAUTION—Federal (U.S.A.) law
prohibits dispensing without
prescription.

0002-5057-68   4   PULL

Calculate the number of ml/dose.
    Pertinent information provided: 250 mg/dose; 125 mg/tsp
    Unit equivalence: 5 ml/tsp
    Desired unit: ml/dose

CORRECT setup:

$$O \times A \times U = Ans$$

$$\frac{250 \text{ mg}}{\text{dose}} \times \frac{\text{tsp}}{125 \text{ mg}} \times \frac{5 \text{ ml}}{\text{tsp}} = 10 \text{ ml/dose}$$

*Ceclor® is a registered trademark of Eli Lilly and Company.

EXAMPLE 6

Ordered: Hydroxyzine syrup 15 mg PO q.i.d.
Available: Atarax syrup 10 mg/5 ml in stock
Calculate the number of tsp/dose.
   Pertinent information provided: 15 mg/dose; 10 mg/5 ml
   Unit equivalency conversion: 5 ml/tsp
   Desired unit: tsp/dose

CORRECT setup:

$$\frac{15 \text{ mg}}{\text{dose}} \times \frac{5 \text{ ml}}{10 \text{ mg}} \times \frac{\text{tsp}}{5 \text{ ml}} = 1.5 \text{ tsp/dose}$$

cc = ml

O × A × U = Ans

EXAMPLE 7

Ordered: 100 kcal/kg per d for a baby who weighs 9 lb 12 oz
Available: Enfamil with iron 20 kcal/fl oz
Calculate the amount in fl oz/d

MINI QUIZ

How do you convert oz to lb?

Answer: Convert with the unit equivalence of 16 oz/lb.

   Pertinent information provided: 100 kcal/kg/d; 20 kcal/fl oz
   Unit equivalency conversion: 16 oz/lb; 2.2 lb/kg
   Desired unit: fl oz/d

CORRECT setup:

1. Convert body weight to lb:

Multiply 12 oz by the conversion factor of 1 lb/16 oz to convert 12 oz to lb. Ans = 0.75 lb. Total body weight in lb – 9 lb + 0.75 lb = 9.75 lb

$$9 \text{ lb} + \left\{ 12 \text{ oz} \times \frac{1 \text{ lb}}{16 \text{ oz}} \right\} = 9.75 \text{ lb}$$

2. Incorporate total body weight (in lb) into the setup:

$$\frac{\text{fl oz}}{20 \text{ kcal}} \times \frac{100 \text{ kcal}}{\text{kg} \cdot \text{d}} \times \frac{\text{kg}}{2.2 \text{ lb}} \times 9.75 \text{ lb} = 22.16 = 22 \text{ fl oz/d}$$

O × A × (body weight) = Ans

You cannot measure 0.16 fl oz. Therefore, round the answer to the nearest measurable unit, that is, 22 fl oz.

EXAMPLE 8

Ordered: Tylenol 5 gr PO q.i.d.
Available: Tylenol elixir 160 mg/tsp
Calculate the dosage in ml/dose.
   Pertinent information provided: 5 gr/dose; 160 mg/tsp
   Unit equivalence: 60 to 65 mg/gr; 5 ml/tsp.
   Desired unit: ml/dose

CORRECT setup:

$$\frac{5 \text{ ml}}{\text{tsp}} \times \frac{\text{tsp}}{160 \text{ mg}} \times \frac{5 \text{ gr}}{\text{dose}} \times \frac{60 \text{ to } 65 \text{ mg}}{1 \text{ gr}} = 9.37 \text{ to } 10.15$$
$$= 9.4 \text{ ml to } 10 \text{ ml/dose}$$

O × U × A × U = Ans

To avoid an overdose, do not round to a higher number.

Round the numbers to the next lowest measurable unit.

You will need a syringe that is calibrated to measure to the 10th of a ml in order to measure 9.4 ml.

Otherwise:

- You will need to round to 9 ml (or use the upper limit of 10 ml).

In a teaspoon:

- 9.4 ml = 1.88 = 1.9 tsp. You will have to round to 1¾ tsp, because you will not be able to measure 1.9 tsp with the available volume of the measuring cup or spoon.

E X A M P L E   9

Ordered: Augmentin 800 mg/d PO in b.i.d. dosage for 10 d
Available: Amoxicillin trihydrate–clavulanate potassium 200 mg/5 ml suspension
Calculate the number of tsp/dose.

M I N I   Q U I Z

What is the problem asking you to do?

Answer: Figure out how many teaspoons of Augmentin you need to give to the patient at each scheduled dose.

Ordered reference dose (Od) = 800 mg/d.
Ordered dose schedule (Os) = b.i.d.

U × A × Od × Os = Ans

Pertinent information provided: 800 mg/d; 2 dose/d; 200 mg/5 ml
Unit equivalency conversion: 5 ml/tsp
Desired unit: tsp/dose

CORRECT setup:

$$\frac{1 \text{ tsp}}{5 \text{ ml}} \times \frac{5 \text{ ml}}{200 \text{ mg}} \times \frac{800 \text{ mg}}{d} \times \frac{d}{2 \text{ dose}} = 2 \text{ tsp/dose}$$

E X A M P L E   1 0

Ordered: Cefaclor 50 mg/kg per d PO q.i.d. for a pediatric patient who weighs 36 lb
Available: Ceclor* 125 mg/5 ml suspension

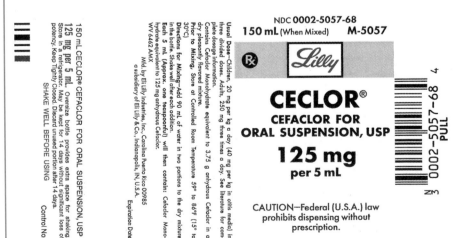

*Ceclor® is a registered trademark of Eli Lilly and Company.

Calculate the number of tsp/dose.

Pertinent information provided: 50 mg/kg per d; 4 dose/d; 125 mg/5 ml; 36 lb

Unit equivalency conversion: 2.2 lb/kg; 5 ml/tsp

Desired unit: tsp/dose

CORRECT setup:

$$36 \; \text{lb} \times \frac{1 \; \text{kg}}{2.2 \; \text{lb}} \times \frac{50 \; \text{mg}}{\text{kg} \cdot \text{d}} \times \frac{\text{d}}{4 \; \text{dose}} \times \frac{5 \; \text{ml}}{125 \; \text{mg}} \times \frac{1 \; \text{tsp}}{5 \; \text{ml}} = 1.6 = 1\tfrac{1}{2} \; \text{tsp/dose}$$

Ordered reference dose (Od) = 50 mg/kg per d. Ordered dose schedule (Os) = q.i.d. = 4 dose/d.

In reality:

BW × U × Od × Os × A × U = Ans

- You will need to round 1.6 tsp to the nearest measurable volume unit of 1½ tsp.
- If you calculate the dosage as ml = 8.18 ml, you can round it to 8 ml and administer the dosage using a 10-ml (cc) syringe.
- If you decide to use a dosage cup (30 cc), you will most likely be able to pour the medication to the 1½ tsp mark, or to approximately 7.5 ml.
- If you are a public health nurse or a home health nurse administering the dosage at the patient's home, and you find a standard 5-ml (1-tsp) dropper, you will first administer 5 ml and then reload with an additional 3 ml to complete this order (5 + 3 = 8 ml).

Large syringes, for example, 20, 30, 60 ml (cc), are not calibrated to measure small volumes, that is, calibration marking with increments of 0.2 ml, 0.25 ml, 0.5 ml, or 1 ml. Therefore, accuracy in volume measurements is limited to the measuring device used.

Frequently, liquid medications use dosage forms in % concentration. Percentage is based on parts per 100 units, for example, 1 part per 100 = 1%; 10 parts per 100 = 10%. The following list shows three possible ways that medications can be mixed to % concentration.

1. % weight/weight, that is, powder diluted with powder:
% medication = gm/100 gm

2. % weight/volume, that is, powder diluted with liquid:
% medication = gm/100 ml

3. % volume/volume, that is, liquid diluted with liquid:
% medication = ml/100 ml

EXAMPLE 1

Ordered: Glucose 10% solution 10 fl oz PO now for a diabetic patient.

Available: A 10-fl oz glass of 10% glucose (gm/ml)

Ten minutes after you have given the glucose solution to the patient, you check the glass and there is 3 fl oz left. Calculate how many gm of glucose has been consumed.

Information provided: 10 fl oz; 10% solution = 10 gm/100 ml; 3 fl oz

Unit equivalence: 30 ml/fl oz

Desired unit: gm

CORRECT setup:

10 fl oz − 3 fl oz = 7 fl oz

$$\frac{10 \; \text{gm}}{100 \; \text{ml}} \times \frac{30 \; \text{ml}}{\text{fl oz}} \times 7 \; \text{fl oz} = 21 \; \text{gm}$$

Read the problem carefully.

Amount consumed = starting volume (vol) − leftover liquid.

Vol consumed × U × A = Ans

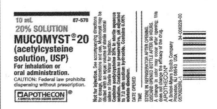

E X A M P L E   2

Ordered: Mucomyst 140 mg/kg for a patient who weighs 106 lb
Available: Acetylcysteine 20% solution (gm/ml)

10 mL   87-570
20% SOLUTION
MUCOMYST®-20
(acetylcysteine
solution, USP)
For inhalation or
oral administration.
CAUTION: Federal law prohibits
dispensing without prescription.
◻APOTHECON®

Calculate the volume in ml necessary for this order.
    Pertinent information provided: 140 mg/kg; 20% = 20 gm/100 ml
    Unit equivalence conversion: 2.2 lb/kg; 1000 mg/gm
    Desired unit: ml

CORRECT setup:

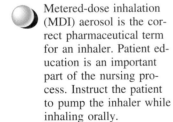

A × U × O × U × BW = Ans

$$\frac{100 \text{ ml}}{20 \text{ gm}} \times \frac{\text{gm}}{1000 \text{ mg}} \times \frac{140 \text{ mg}}{\text{kg}} \times \frac{1 \text{ kg}}{2.2 \text{ lb}} \times 106 \text{ lb} = 33.7 \text{ ml}$$

In reality:

- If you use a medication dosage cup to measure this dose, you will most likely round 33.7 ml to 30 ml.
- If you take the time to use two 20-ml (cc) syringes to measure, you will be able to measure this dose at either 33 ml (20 + 13) or 34 ml (20 + 14).

    In either case, you will not be able to measure 33.7 ml precisely.

Take note of the increments in the calibration marks on the syringe, for example, 0.1, 0.2, 0.25, 0.5, 1, 5, 10 ml.

Metered-dose inhalation (MDI) aerosol is the correct pharmaceutical term for an inhaler. Patient education is an important part of the nursing process. Instruct the patient to pump the inhaler while inhaling orally.

If your patient needs a spacer and does not have one handy, he or she can use the hollow cardboard core from a roll of toilet tissue.

Inhaler and Spray Pumps

You need to provide instruction to the patient on the proper use of inhalers. Effective inhalation is essential for the medication to reach the bronchial tree in order to provide optimal efficacy. Encourage patients to use spacers, for example, the Aerochamber or Inspirease, in order to achieve effective delivery of medication to the airway.

    Improper use of an inhaler causes the medication to spray into the mouth; subsequently, the medication is swallowed, producing undesirable side effects.

E X A M P L E   1

    Ordered: Proventil metered-dose 2 puffs PO inhalation q.i.d.
    Available: Proventil Inhalation Aerosol 90 µg/puff
Calculate the dosage in µg/dose.
    Pertinent information provided: 2 puff/dose; 90 µg/puff
    Unit equivalency conversion: None needed
    Desired unit: µg/dose

A × O = Ans

CORRECT setup:

$$\frac{90 \text{ µg}}{\text{puff}} \times \frac{2 \text{ puff}}{\text{dose}} = 180 \text{ µg/dose}$$

EXAMPLE   2

Ordered: Cromolyn sodium 20 mg inhaled q.i.d.
Available: Cromolyn sodium 20 mg inhaler capsule
Calculate the number of capsule/dose.
Pertinent information provided: 20 mg/dose; 20 mg/capsule
Unit equivalency conversion: None needed
Desired unit: Capsule (cap)

CORRECT setup:

$$\frac{20 \text{ mg}}{\text{dose}} \times \frac{\text{cap}}{20 \text{ mg}} = 1 \text{ cap}$$

Cromolyn contained in a capsule is prepared for inhalation by placing the capsule in a mechanism called a Rotocap. This device cuts the capsule open to release the powdered medication for inhalation.

O × A = Ans

EXAMPLE   3

Ordered: Vancenase AQ (DS) nasal 84 μg each nostril (1 spray each nostril) q.h.s.
Available: Vancenase AQ (DS) (beclomethasone dipropionate) nasal spray 0.084% (dry weight), 12.5 gm/bottle
Calculate the number of sprays/bottle.
Pertinent information provided: 84 μg/spray;
0.084% = 0.084 gm/100 gm; 12.5 gm/bottle
Unit equivalency conversion: 1,000,000 μg/gm
Desired unit: sprays/bottle

Aqueous (AQ) solutions are delivered by manual pump and are also available in aerosol form.

CORRECT setup:

$$\frac{1}{\cancel{12.5 \text{ gm}}} \times \frac{\overset{125,000}{\cancel{\underset{250,000}{1,000,000}}} \text{ μg}}{\text{gm}} \times \frac{0.001}{\underset{4}{100 \text{ gm}}} \times \frac{\text{spray}}{\underset{2}{84 \text{ μg}}} = 125 \text{ sprays/bottle}$$

To decrease irritation after administration of a nasal spray, point the tip of the nozzle away from the patient; instruct the patient to do likewise.

A × U × A × O = Ans

CALCULATIONS FOR ADMINISTRATION OF TOPICAL MEDICATIONS

Dosage Form	Definition
Lotions	Semiliquid preparations of medication for topical application. A lotion can be either water- or oil-based.
Creams	Water-based semisolid preparations of medication for topical application.
Ointments	Oil-based semisolid preparations of medication for topical application.
Pastes	Semisolid preparations of medication with adhesive properties for topical application.
Patches	Adhesive materials with medication placed in center; the adhesive materials allow secure placement for absorption of medication on the skin over a long period of time.

Diluent. A medium for decreasing the medication concentration, such as water, alcohol, petroleum gel.

Write down all the units in the question to avoid any error in the placement of the conversion factor.

0.05% wet weight (w/w) = 0.05 gm/100 gm

U × O = Ans

Answer: Calculate the midpoint of a week.

You know the midpoint of a week is 3.5 d.

Ordered dose schedule (Os) = Two dose/week

U × Os = time to next dose

To administer Nitro-Bid, measure 1 inch of ointment onto the Appli-Ruler section of the Appli-Tape. Spread the ointment carefully by folding the Appli-Tape. Remove the outer, lined section of the adhesive border, and press it firmly to the skin.

A × O = Ans

The amount of medication contained in lotions, ointments, creams, pastes, or patches is a relative % concentration of medication in a diluent. The following are examples of topical dosage calculations.

EXAMPLE 1

Ordered: Psorcon 0.05% cream q.d., applied thinly to affected area
Available: Diflorasone diacetate 0.05% cream
Convert dosage to mg/100 gm.
Pertinent information provided: 0.05% = 0.05 gm/100 gm dose
Unit equivalency conversion: 1000 mg/gm
Desired unit: gm Psorcon/100 gm dose

CORRECT setup:

$$\frac{1000 \text{ mg}}{\text{gm}} \times \frac{0.05 \text{ gm Psorcon}}{100 \text{ gm dose}} = 50 \text{ mg/100 gm dose}$$

Answer: .05 gm/100 gm dose

EXAMPLE 2

Ordered: Estraderm 0.05 mg/d patch apply twice weekly
Available: Estraderm (estradiol) 0.05 mg/d patch.
Your patient has applied her first patch at 9:00 AM Monday morning. She asks you when will she need to apply the second patch.

MINI QUIZ

What is the problem asking you to do?

Pertinent information provided: 2 dose/wk
Unit equivalency conversion: 7 d/wk
Desired unit: d/dose (or to the next dose)

CORRECT setup:

$$\frac{7 \text{ d}}{\text{wk}} \times \frac{\text{wk}}{2 \text{ dose}} = 3.5 \text{ d to the next dose}$$

Answer: 3.5 d from 9:00 AM Monday = 9:00 PM Thursday

EXAMPLE 3

Ordered: Nitro-Bid 2% ointment, 1 inch ointment topical q.6hr to upper arm
Available: Nitrol (nitroglycerin) 2% ointment and appli-kit
Calculate the dosage in mg of nitroglycerin/dose (1 inch ointment = 15 mg nitroglycerin).
Pertinent information provided: 1 inch/dose; 15 mg Nitrol/1 inch oint
Unit equivalency conversion: None needed
Desired unit: mg Nitrol/dose.

CORRECT setup:

$$\frac{15 \text{ mg Nitrol}}{1 \text{ inch oint}} \times \frac{1 \text{ inch}}{\text{dose}} = 15 \text{ mg Nitrol/dose}$$

EXAMPLE   4

Ordered: Differin 0.1% (w/w) gel apply q.h.s. to skin eruptions
Available: Differin (adapalene) 0.1% gel

Calculate dosage in mg/gm.

Pertinent information provided: 0.1% = 0.1 gm Differin/100 gm gel
Unit equivalency conversion: 1000 mg/gm
Desired unit: mg Differin/gm gel

CORRECT setup:

$$\frac{0.1 \ \cancel{gm} \text{ Differin}}{100 \text{ gm gel}} \times \frac{1000 \text{ mg}}{\cancel{gm}} = 1 \text{ mg Differin/gm gel}$$

 % w/w = gm medication per 100 gm diluent.

 A × U = Ans

CALCULATIONS FOR ADMINISTRATION OF EAR AND EYE DROPS

Medications to be instilled into the ears or eyes are available in the dosage forms of solutions and suspensions. Orders for medication dosages are based on the number of drops (gtt) to be administered to a specific site, for example, the eyes (OS, left; OD, right; OU, left and right), and the ears (AS, left; AD, right; AU, left and right). Always check the meaning of the abbreviations with the provider prior to administration, for example, left eye, right eye, both eyes.

To ensure uniformity of drop size in the administration of ear and eye drops, you need to hold the dropper perpendicular to the site of instillation. Holding the dropper at a slanted angle increases the size of the drop and thereby increases the medication dosage. Additionally, you will need to instruct the patient to blink lightly after instillation to keep the medication within the conjunctival sac.

After instillation of ear drops, you will need to instruct the patient to keep his or her head tilted for approximately 3 to 5 min to allow sufficient time for medication to flow into the ear canal. Also, if you place a cotton ball lightly over the ear canal, you can prevent medication from discharging onto the patient's shoulder.

The following are examples of dosage calculation problems using ear and eye medications.

 0.01% = 0.01 gm/100 ml
OU = both eyes

EXAMPLE   1

Ordered: Decadron 0.01% ophth solution 2 gtt OU q.i.d.
Available: Dexamethasone 0.01% ophthalmic solution

Calculate mg/dose of dexamethasone ordered (15 gtt/ml).

Pertinent information provided: 0.01%; 2 gtt/eye; 2 eyes/dose; 15 gtt/ml
Unit equivalency conversion: 1000 mg/gm
Desired unit: mg/dose

CORRECT setup:

$$\frac{1000 \text{ mg}}{\cancel{gm}} \times \frac{0.01 \ \cancel{gm}}{100 \ \cancel{ml}} \times \frac{1 \ \cancel{ml}}{15 \ \cancel{gtt}} \times \frac{2 \ \cancel{gtt}}{\cancel{eye}} \times \frac{2 \ \cancel{eye}}{\text{dose}} = 0.0266 = 0.027 \text{ mg/dose}$$

 The order is 2 gtt/eye per dose. Therefore gtt/dose = 4 gtt/dose, that is,

$$\frac{2 \text{ gtt}}{\cancel{eye} \cdot \text{dose}} \times 2 \ \cancel{eyes} = 4 \text{ gtt/dose}$$

 U × A × U × O × O = Ans

EXAMPLE 2

Ordered: Ciprofloxacin HCl 0.3% ophth solution 2 gtt OU q.i.d. for 7 d
Available: Ciloxan ophthalmic drops 2.5 ml (15 gtt/ml)

CAUTION: FEDERAL (USA) LAW PROHIBITS DISPENSING
WITHOUT PRESCRIPTION.
FOR TOPICAL OPHTHALMIC USE ONLY.
INGREDIENTS: Each mL contains: Active: Ciprofloxacin HCl
3.5 mg equivalent to 3 mg base. Preservative: Benzalkonium
Chloride 0.006%. Inactive: Sodium Acetate, Acetic Acid,
Mannitol, Edetate Disodium, Hydrochloric Acid and/or Sodium
Hydroxide (to adjust pH) and Purified Water.   DM-00
USUAL DOSAGE: Read enclosed insert.
STORAGE: Store at 2° to 30°C (36° to 86°F).
U.S. Patent No. 4,670,444.
ALCON LABORATORIES, INC.
Fort Worth, Texas 76134 USA
Printed in USA

UNIT OF USE
NDC 0065-0656-25 **Alcon®**
Ciloxan®
(Ciprofloxacin HCl)
0.3% as base
Ophthalmic
Solution
Sterile 2.5 mL

LOT: EXP: 320063-0395

Do you have enough medication for this order?

Key: O = 4 gtt/dose. Os = q.i.d. Ot = 7 d.

Pertinent information provided: 4 gtt/dose; 4 dose/d; 7d; 15 gtt/ml
Unit equivalency conversion: None needed
Desired unit: ml

CORRECT setup:

Key: U × O × Os × Ot = Ans

$$\frac{1 \text{ ml}}{15 \text{ gtt}} \times \frac{4 \text{ gtt}}{\text{dose}} \times \frac{4 \text{ dose}}{\text{d}} \times 7 \text{ d} = 7.5 \text{ ml}$$

Answer: 2.5 ml < 7.5 ml. No, there is not enough.

Key: You will need three bottles to complete this order.

EXAMPLE 3

Ordered: Alomide 0.1% ophth solution 2 gtt OU q4hr.
Available: Alomide (lodoxamide tromethamine) 0.1% ophthalmic solution 10 ml bottle (15 gtt/ml)

CAUTION: FEDERAL (USA) LAW PROHIBITS DISPENSING
WITHOUT PRESCRIPTION. EACH mL CONTAINS: Lodoxamide
Tromethamine 1.78 mg, equivalent to 1 mg Lodoxamide.
STORAGE: Store at 15-27°C (59-80°F).
FOR TOPICAL OPHTHALMIC USE ONLY.
USUAL DOSAGE: Instill one to two drops in affected eye(s)
four times daily.
ALCON LABORATORIES, INC., Fort Worth, Texas 76134 USA

NDC 0065-0345-10 **Alcon®**
Alomide® 0.1%
(Lodoxamide
Tromethamine
Ophthalmic
Solution) Sterile 10 mL

LOT: EXP: 248673-0595

Calculate the number of μg of medication per dose.

MINI QUIZ

What is the problem asking you to do?

Answer: To calculate the dosage in μg/dose.

Pertinent information provided: 0.1% = 0.1 gm/100 ml; 4 gtt/dose; 15 gtt/ml
Unit equivalency conversion: 1000 mg/gm; 1000 μg/mg (1,000,000 μg/gm)
Desired unit: μg/dose

Key: You can use 1,000,000 μg/gm and eliminate another step in your setup.

CORRECT setup:

Key: U × A × U × O = Ans

$$\frac{1000 \text{ μg}}{\text{mg}} \times \frac{1000 \text{ mg}}{\text{gm}} \times \frac{0.1 \text{ gm}}{100 \text{ ml}} \times \frac{1 \text{ ml}}{15 \text{ gtt}} \times \frac{4 \text{ gtt}}{\text{dose}} = 266.666 = 266.7 \text{ μg/dose}$$

EXAMPLE 4

Ordered: Cortisporin otic drops 4 gtt AU q.i.d. for 10 d
Available: Cortisporin (hydrocortisone; neomycin sulfate; polymyxin B sulfate) otic suspension 15 ml (15 gtt/ml)
Is 15 ml of Cortisporin suspension enough for this order?
   Pertinent information provided: 8 gtt/dose; 4 dose/d; 10d; 15 ml; 15 gtt/ml
   Unit equivalency conversion: None needed
   Desired unit: ml

CORRECT setup:

$$\frac{1 \text{ ml}}{15 \text{ gtt}} \times \frac{8 \text{ gtt}}{\text{dose}} \times \frac{4 \text{ dose}}{\text{d}} \times 10 \text{ d} = 21.3 \text{ ml}$$

Answer: 15 ml < 21.3 ml. No, there is not enough.

 AU indicates both ears. Correct abbreviations are an important part of the safety canon.

 This case is similar to example 1; you will need 4 gtt for each ear; a total of 8 drops/dose.

 U × O × Os × Ot = Ans

EXAMPLE 5

Ordered: Maxitrol ophth suspension 2 gtt OU b.i.d.
Available: Maxitrol ophthalmic solution 15-ml vial

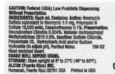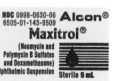

Calculate the number of dose/vial (15 gtt/ml).
   Pertinent information provided: 4 gtt/dose; 2 dose/d; 5 ml
   Unit equivalency conversion: 15 gtt/ml
   Desired unit: dose/vial

CORRECT setup:

$$\frac{\text{dose}}{4 \text{ gtt}} \times \frac{15 \text{ gtt}}{\text{ml}} \times \frac{5 \text{ ml}}{\text{vial}} = 18.7 \text{ dose/vial}$$
$$= 18 \text{ dose/vial}$$

 This is not a typical question; it is, rather, a test of your analytical abilities and math skills.

 Gently shake the bottle prior to administering medication in suspension.

 A × U × O × Os = Ans

CALCULATIONS FOR ADMINISTRATION OF SUPPOSITORIES, ENEMAS, AND IRRIGATIONS

Dosage Form	Definition
Suppositories	Mixtures of medication plus a diluent, which melt at body temperature. A suppository (supp) is specially shaped for easy insertion into a designated body cavity.
Enemas and irrigations	Solutions of medications dissolved in a large quantity of water, available in ready-to-use preparations. Whenever the ready-to-use dosage form is not available, dilution of a stock solution will be necessary prior to administration of the enema or irrigation.

The following are examples of dosage calculations used in administering suppositories, enemas, and ready-to-use solutions.

Rectal suppositories are clearly labeled for rectal administration.

> ### E X A M P L E   1
>
> **Ordered:** Promethazine HCl 25 mg PR t.i.d. p.r.n.
> **Available:** Phenergan 12.5-mg suppositories

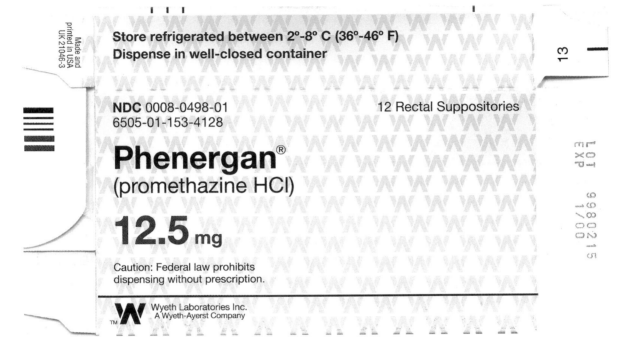

Store refrigerated between 2°-8° C (36°-46° F)
Dispense in well-closed container

13

NDC 0008-0498-01
6505-01-153-4128

12 Rectal Suppositories

Phenergan®
(promethazine HCl)

12.5 mg

Caution: Federal law prohibits dispensing without prescription.

W Wyeth Laboratories Inc.
A Wyeth-Ayerst Company
TM

Made and printed in USA
UK 21046-3

LOT
EXP

9980215
1/00

Rectal suppositories administered vaginally by error (route error) cause secondary burns.

O × A = Ans

Calculate the number of suppositories/dose.
   Pertinent information provided: 25 mg/dose; 12.5-mg suppository
   Unit equivalency conversion: None needed
   Desired unit: supp

CORRECT setup:

$$\frac{25 \text{ mg}}{\text{dose}} \times \frac{\text{supp}}{12.5 \text{ mg}} = 2 \text{ supp}$$

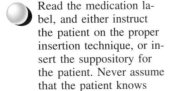

Read the medication label, and either instruct the patient on the proper insertion technique, or insert the suppository for the patient. Never assume that the patient knows what needs to be done.

A True Story
A patient was given a rectal suppository for insertion, but swallowed it instead.

Another True Story
When given a rectal suppository still in its full wrapper, the patient inserted it without removing the wrapper.

EXAMPLE 2

Ordered: Clotrimazole vaginal tab 500 mg q.h.s. single dose
Available: Clotrimazole 500-mg vaginal tab
Calculate the number of tab/dose.
Pertinent information provided: 500 mg/dose; 500 mg/tab
Unit equivalency conversion: None needed
Desired unit: tab

CORRECT setup:

$$\frac{500 \text{ mg}}{\text{dose}} \times \frac{\text{tab}}{500 \text{ mg}} = 1 \text{ tab/dose}$$

EXAMPLE 3

Ordered: Hydrocortisone enema PR q.h.s. for 3 nights
Available: Hydrocortisone 100 mg/60 ml enema
Calculate the dosage of hydrocortisone % solution.
Pertinent information provided: 100 mg/60 ml
Unit equivalency conversion: 1000 mg/gm
Desired unit: gm/100 ml

CORRECT setup:

$$\frac{100 \text{ mg}}{60 \text{ ml}} \times \frac{\text{gm}}{1000 \text{ mg}} \times 100 = 0.166 \text{ (gm/100 ml)} = 0.17\% \text{ solution}$$

 Vaginal tablets are labeled for their route of administration, and they are specially shaped for intravaginal application.

 O × A = Ans

 % concentration (w/v) = gm/100 ml.

 A × U × % solution = Ans

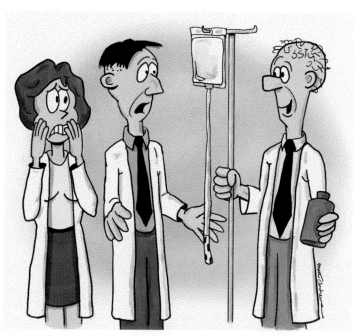

"JIM, I'M GIVING MR. TAYLOR HIS CITRATE OF MAGNESIA NOW!"

Enema and Irrigation Solutions From Stock Solutions

A stock solution is a standard concentration of medication in solution that is available in stock or store. Dilution is the process of adding water to decrease the concentration of the available stock solution. When a ready-to-use preparation is not available, it may be up to the nurse to make the solution from available powdered (or crystalline) medications, or a stock solution as ordered for administration.

The following rules can be applied to the calculation of dosage problems on the dilution of a stock solution:

1. Start with the ordered concentration (Oc), for example, 0.9 gm/100 ml (w/v), 10 ml/100 ml (v/v), 25 gm/100 gm (w/w).
2. Carry out the appropriate unit conversion steps that will show you the desired unit dimension, for example, ml to L, mg to kg, μg to mg.
3. Place the ordered volume (Ov) next, for example, 0.5 L, 1 kg.
4. Carry out the appropriate unit conversion steps to find the desired unit dimension.
5. Place the available concentration (Ac) and/or the available volume (Av) next, that is, the concentration of the stock solution and/or the volume of the stock solution.

The following are dosage calculation problems on the dilution of stock solutions.

Normal saline is a stock solution of 0.9% sodium chloride (NaCl) solution, that is, 0.9 gm NaCl in 100 ml water.

The ordered concentration is:
Oc = 0.9 gm/100 ml.

The ordered volume is:
Ov = 0.5 L/dose.

Oc × U × Ov = Answer

EXAMPLE   1

Ordered: Normal saline 0.5 L enema stat
Available: Sodium chloride crystals
Calculate the amount of sodium chloride in gm needed to make 0.5 L of solution.
Pertinent information provided: 0.5 L/dose normal saline = 0.9% = water; 0.9 gm/100 ml
Unit equivalency conversion: 1000 ml/1 L
Desired unit: gm sodium chloride/dose

CORRECT setup:

$$\frac{0.9 \text{ gm}}{100 \text{ ml}} \times \frac{1000 \text{ ml}}{1 \text{ L}} \times \frac{0.5 \text{ L}}{\text{dose}} = 4.5 \text{ gm}$$

Ordered concentration × Unit equiv conversion × Ordered volume = Answer

EXAMPLE   2

Ordered: Neosporin 1% solution 4 L for urinary bladder irrigation
Available: Neosporin 5-gm tablets
Calculate the number of gm of Neosporin necessary for this order.
Pertinent information provided: 1% = 1 gm/100 ml water; 4 L/dose; 5 gm/tab
Unit equivalency conversion: 1000 ml/1 L
Desired unit: tab Neosporin/dose

Oc = 1 gm/100 ml
Ov = 4 L/dose

CORRECT setup:

$$\frac{1 \text{ gm}}{100 \text{ ml}} \times \frac{1000 \text{ ml}}{1 \text{ L}} \times \frac{4 \text{ L}}{\text{dose}} \times \frac{\text{tab}}{5 \text{ gm}} = 8 \text{ tab/dose}$$

Ordered   ×   Unit equiv   ×   Ordered   ×   Available   =   Answer
concentration   conversion   volume   concentration

 Oc × U × Ov × Ac = Ans

E X A M P L E   3

Ordered: Clorox (bleach) solution 1% 2 L for surface sanitizing
Available: Clorox (hypochlorous acid) 7% stock solution
Calculate the amount of stock solution in ml needed for this order.
Pertinent information provided: 1% = 1 ml bleach/100 ml ordered;
　　2 L/dose; 7% = 7 ml bleach/100 ml stock
Unit equivalency conversion: 1000 ml/1 L
Desired unit: ml stock solution/dose

 Ov = 2 L

CORRECT setup:

$$\frac{1 \text{ ml bleach}}{100 \text{ ml}} \times \frac{1000 \text{ ml}}{1 \text{ L}} \times \frac{2 \text{ L}}{\text{dose}} \times \frac{100 \text{ ml stock}}{7 \text{ ml bleach}} = 285.7 \text{ ml stock/dose}$$

Ordered   ×   Unit equiv   ×   Ordered   ×   Available   =   Answer
concentration   conversion   volume   concentration

 Oc × U × Ov × Av = Ans

To make this solution, mix approximately 280 ml of 7% bleach in 1720 ml of water. You will need a beaker or measuring cylinder to measure the stock solution. Transfer the stock solution to a 2-L container and add water.

 It will be difficult to measure 285.7 = 286 ml exactly to the ml without a measuring cylinder. Most likely, you will mix 280 ml of stock with 1720 ml water.

E X A M P L E   4

Ordered: Hydrogen peroxide 1.5% 500 ml to clean a laceration wound measuring 5 cm
Available: Hydrogen peroxide 3% stock solution
Calculate the amount of stock solution in (ml needed) for this order.
Pertinent information provided: 1.5% = 1.5 ml peroxide/100 ml;
　　500 ml/dose; 3% = 3 ml peroxide/100 ml stock
Unit equivalency conversion: None needed
Desired unit: ml 3% peroxide/dose

 Start the setup with the ordered concentration and set up the rest of the conversion factors to allow unit cancellation.

 Oc = 1.5% = 1.5 ml/ 100 ml. Ov = 500 ml. Av = 3% = 3 ml/100 ml

CORRECT setup:

$$\frac{1.5 \text{ ml peroxide}}{100 \text{ ml}} \times \frac{500 \text{ ml}}{\text{dose}} \times \frac{100 \text{ ml stock}}{3 \text{ ml peroxide}} = 250 \text{ ml stock/dose}$$

Ordered   ×   Ordered   ×   Available
concentration   volume   concentration

 Oc × Ov × Av = Ans

Dilution of Stock Solution for Miscellaneous Applications

An order for the dilution of a stock solution can be written in ratio format. A dilution ratio is a mathematical ratio employed to express the proportionality between the substrate and the diluent. For example, a 1:10 dilution of a solution requires that you add 10 parts of the diluent to 1 part of the substrate or original concentrate. You can substitute any type of unit dimension to

Part = any dimension in weight or volume measurements, for example,

$$1:1 = \frac{1 \text{ fl oz peroxide}}{1 \text{ fl oz water}} \quad \text{or}$$

$$\frac{1 \text{ ml peroxide}}{1 \text{ ml water}} \quad \text{or}$$

$$\frac{1 \text{ gm peroxide}}{1 \text{ gm water}}$$

The following setup is used to calculate the amount of the stock solution you will need for dilution.

Volume of stock solution = dilution (D) × ordered volume (Ov).

D = 1:10 = 1 ml Clorox/ 10 part water.
Ov = 500 ml

D × Ov = Ans

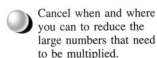

Cancel when and where you can to reduce the large numbers that need to be multiplied.

Ordered concentration (Oc) = 10% = 10 in 100 = 10 parts boric acid/100 parts water
Ordered volume (Ov) = 2 L
Available concentration (Ac) = 40% = 40 ml boric acid/100 ml

Oc × Ov × U × Ac = Ans

represent the "part" as long as the part and the unit dimension are equivalent, for example, 1 ml of concentrate to 1 ml of water.

Review Chapter 1 if you have any difficulty with ratios, fractions, or percentages. The following are examples of stock solution dilution problems that are based on ratios.

E X A M P L E   1

Ordered: Hypochlorous acid 1 : 10 solution 500 ml
Available: Clorox liquid
Calculate the amount of Clorox liquid necessary to make this solution.
    Pertinent information provided: 1 : 10 dilution; 500 ml/dose
    Unit equivalency conversion: None needed
    Desired unit: ml Clorox liquid/dose

CORRECT setup:

$$\underset{\text{Ordered dilution}}{\frac{1 \text{ ml Clorox}}{10 \text{ ml}}} \times \underset{\text{Ordered volume}}{\frac{500 \text{ ml}}{\text{dose}}} = \underset{\text{Answer}}{50 \text{ ml Clorox/dose}}$$

Place 50 ml Clorox in a container and add water to a total volume of 500 ml, that is, 450 ml water.

E X A M P L E   2

Ordered: boric acid 10% solution 2 L
Available: boric acid 40% stock solution
Calculate the amount of stock solution in ml necessary for this order.
    Pertinent information provided: 10% = 10 ml boric acid/100 ml water = 1 ml/10 ml; 40% = 40 gm/100 ml stock; 2 L/dose
    Unit equivalency conversion: 1000 ml/L
    Desired unit: ml stock solution/dose.

CORRECT setup:

$$\underset{\substack{\text{Ordered}\\\text{concentration}}}{\frac{1 \text{ ml boric acid}}{10 \text{ ml}}} \times \underset{\substack{\text{Ordered}\\\text{volume}}}{\frac{2 \text{ L}}{\text{dose}}} \times \underset{\substack{\text{Unit equiv}\\\text{concentration}}}{\frac{1000 \text{ ml}}{1 \text{ L}}} \times \underset{\substack{\text{Available}\\\text{concentration}}}{\frac{100 \text{ ml stock}}{40 \text{ ml boric acid}}} = 500 \text{ ml stock/dose}$$

E X A M P L E   3

Ordered: Betadine 1 : 10 dilution, to make 1 L.
Available: Betadine 10% stock solution

NDC 0034-2100-01
NSN 6505-00-754-0374

BETADINE solution *povidone-iodine,10%**

For Professional and Hospital Use Only Not Labeled for Consumer Use

Topical Antiseptic Bactericide/ Virucide for Degerming Skin and Mucous Membranes

One Gallon (3.78 liters)

FOR PROFESSIONAL AND HOSPITAL USE ONLY

BETADINE solution
TOPICAL ANTISEPTIC BACTERICIDE/VIRUCIDE
Kills gram-positive and gram-negative bacteria, viruses, fungi, protozoa and yeasts. Film-forming, virtually nonirritating and nonstaining to skin and natural fabrics.
Directions: Apply BETADINE Solution full strength as often as needed as a paint, wet soak or spray.
Kills pathogens in primary or secondary topical infections, surgical incisions, decubitis or stasis ulcers, traumatic lesions and first-, second- and third-degree burns. Use prophylactically to help prevent

microbial contamination. May be covered with gauze or adhesive bandage.
Warnings: For External Use Only. In preoperative prepping, avoid "pooling" beneath the patient. Prolonged exposure to wet solution may cause irritation or rarely, severe skin reactions. In rare instance of local irritation or sensitivity, discontinue use. Do not heat prior to application.
AVOID STORING AT EXCESSIVE HEAT.
Inactive Ingredients: Citric acid, Dibasic sodium phosphate, Glycerin, and other ingredients.
*equal to 1% available iodine

THE PURDUE FREDERICK COMPANY, NORWALK, CT 06850-3590
M7968 L97

Calculate the amount of Betadine stock solution (in ml) for this order.

M I N I   Q U I Z

Is the information about the stock concentration pertinent?

Pertinent information provided: $1:10$ = 1 ml of Betadine stock/10 ml of water; 1 L/dose
Unit equivalency conversion: 1000 ml/L
Desired unit: ml Betadine stock solution

CORRECT setup:

$$\frac{1 \text{ ml Betadine stock}}{10 \text{ ml}} \times \frac{1 \text{ L}}{\text{dose}} \times \frac{1000 \text{ ml}}{1 \text{ L}} = 100 \text{ ml Betadine stock/dose}$$

Answer: No. You are simply making a 1-to-10 dilution of the stock solution.

Oc = Ordered concentration = $1:10$ = 1 part Betadine/10 parts water
Ov = ordered volume = 1 L

Oc × Ov × U = Ans

E X A M P L E   4

Ordered: Cetylcide $1:64$ solution 1 gal
Available: Cetylcide stock solution
Calculate in fl oz the volume of Cetylcide stock solution needed for this order.

M I N I   Q U I Z

What is the problem asking you to do?

Pertinent information provided: $1:64$ = 1 part Cetylcide/64 parts water; 1 gal/dose
Unit equivalency conversion: 128 fl oz/gal
Desired unit: fl oz Cetylcide stock/dose

CORRECT setup:

$$\frac{1 \text{ fl oz Cetylcide}}{64 \text{ fl oz}} \times \frac{1 \text{ gal}}{\text{dose}} \times \frac{128 \text{ fl oz}}{1 \text{ gal}} = 2 \text{ fl oz stock/dose}$$

Answer: Make 1 gal of $1:64$ dilution of the stock solution.

Ordered concentration (Oc) = $1:64$ = 1 fl oz/64 fl oz
Ordered volume = 1 gallon

Oc × Ov × U = Ans

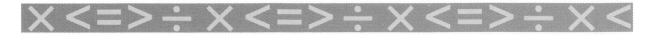

Chapter Summary

If you are having any problems understanding the implementation process of DA, please review Chapters 3 and 4 again. The following list is an approach that students may use to solve dosage calculation problems:

✔ Read and interpret the problem carefully to determine what you are being asked to solve.
✔ Always place the dimension units next to their corresponding numbers—do not take short cuts.
✔ Follow the steps outlined in Chapter 3 to extract pertinent information from the problem.

✔ Follow the steps outlined under each dosage form section in this chapter, for example, diluting solution, % concentration conversion, diluting from stock.
✔ Remember that your desired unit dimension must be kept in its proper place, so that all unwanted units can be canceled.
✔ Always recheck your math. No amount of DA can rectify poor math skills.
✔ Review Chapter 1 if you still have problems with percentages and ratios.

PROBLEM SET	PROBLEM SET ANSWERS

1. Ordered: Amoxil 500 mg PO t.i.d.
     Available: Amoxicillin 250-mg capsule
     Calculate the number of cap/dose.
	1. 2 cap

2. Ordered: Captopril 50 mg q.d.
     Available: Captopril 12.5-mg tab
     Calculate the number of tab/dose.
	2. 4 tab

3. Ordered: Docusate 100 mg PO t.i.d.
     Available: Docusate sodium 100-mg gelcap
     Calculate the number of cap/d.
	3. 3 cap

PROBLEM SET	PROBLEM SET ANSWERS

4. Ordered: Flagyl 500 mg PO b.i.d.
   Available: Flagyl (metronidazole HCl) 250-mg tab
   Calculate the number of tab/dose.

   4. 2 tab

5. Ordered: Proventil liquid 4 mg PO t.i.d.
   Available: Proventil (albuterol sulfate) liquid 2 mg/tsp
   Calculate the number of ml/dose.

   5. 10 ml

6. Ordered: Ciloxan ophth 2 gtt OS q.3hr
   Available: Ciloxan (ciprofloxacin) ophthalmic solution
   Calculate dosage in mg/gtt. Use unit equivalence 15 gtt/ml.

   6. 10 mg/gtt

7. Ordered: Ambien 2.5 mg q.h.s.
   Available: Ambien (zolpidem tartrate) 5 mg-tab
   Calculate the number of tab/dose.

   7. ½ tab

8. Ordered: Betadine 2% solution 1 L
   Available: Betadine (povidone-iodine) 10% stock solution
   Calculate (in ml) the amount of Betadine stock solution needed for this order.

   8. 200-ml stock solution

P R O B L E M S E T	PROBLEM SET ANSWERS
9. Ordered: Sodium chloride 0.45% solution, 500 ml Available: Sodium chloride crystals Calculate (in mg) the amount of sodium chloride needed for this order.	9. 2250 mg
10. Ordered: Hydrogen peroxide 1 : 5 dilution, 2 L Available: Hydrogen peroxide 3% stock solution Calculate (in ml) the amount of stock solution needed for this order.	10. 400-ml stock solution
11. Ordered: Ceclor 325 mg PO t.i.d. Available: Ceclor (cefaclor) 125 mg/5 ml suspension Calculate the number of tsp/dose.	11. 2⅔ tsp
12. Ordered: Zyrtec liquid 10 mg PO q.d. Available: Zyrtec (cetirizine HCl) liquid 5 mg/tsp Calculate the number of tsp/dose.	12. 2 tsp
13. Ordered: Cedax 150 mg PO q.d. Available: Cedax (ceftibuten) 90 mg/tsp suspension Calculate the number of ml/dose.	13. 8.3 ml = 8 ml

PROBLEM SET	PROBLEM SET ANSWERS

14. Ordered: Kenalog 0.1% cream top q.h.s.
Available: Kenalog (triamcinolone acetonide) 0.1% cream
(0.1 gm/100 gm)
Calculate the number of mg/gm.

14. 1 mg/gm

15. Ordered: Biaxin 150 mg PO b.i.d.
Available: Clarithromycin 250 mg/tsp
Calculate the number of ml/dose.

15. 3 ml/dose

16. Ordered: Hytrin 4 mg PO q.h.s.
Available: Hytrin (terazosin HCl) 2 mg/capsule
Calculate the number of cap/dose.

16. 2 cap/dose

17. Ordered: K-Dur 20 mg PO q.d.
Available: K-Dur (potassium chloride) 10-mg tab
Calculate the number of tab/dose.

17. 2 tab/dose

PROBLEM SET	PROBLEM SET ANSWERS

28. Ordered: Prilosec 20 mg PO b.i.d.
     Available: Prilosec (omeprazole) 10-mg capsule
     Calculate the number of cap/d.
	28. 4 cap/d

29. Ordered: Zantac 300 mg PO b.i.d.
     Available: Ranitidine HCl 15 mg/ml syrup
     Calculate the number of tsp/dose.
	29. 4 tsp/dose

30. Ordered: Cipro 500 mg PO b.i.d. for 2 wk
     Available: Cipro (ciprofloxacin) 500-mg tab
     Calculate the number of tab/d.
	30. 2 tab/d

31. Ordered: Voltaren 50 mg PO t.i.d.
     Available: Voltaren (diclofenac sodium) 25-mg tab
     Calculate the number of tab/dose.
	31. 2 tab/dose

32. Ordered: EtOH 10% 1 pt
     Available: EtOH 95% stock solution 1 pt.
     Calculate the number of ml of EtOH stock solution for this order.
	32. 50.5 ml or 50 ml of
	        EtOH stock solution.

PROBLEM SET	PROBLEM SET ANSWERS
33. Convert 20% glucose solution into mg/ml.	33. 200 mg/ml
34. Ordered: NS 1 L solution (NS = 0.9%) Available: NaCl crystals Calculate the number of mg of NaCl needed to fill this order.	34. 9000 mg
35. Ordered: Relafen 500 mg PO b.i.d. Available: Relafen (nabumetone) 500 mg Calculate the number of gm/dose.	35. 0.5 gm/dose
36. Ordered: Norvasc 10 mg PO q.d. Available: Norvasc (amlodipine) 2.5-mg tab Calculate the number of tab/dose.	36. 4 tab/dose
37. Ordered: Capoten 150 mg PO t.i.d. Available: Captopril 12.5-mg, 25-mg, 50-mg, and 100-mg tab Which of the available dosage forms would require the least amount of effort for administration?	37. Three 50-mg tab, preferably one 100-mg and one 50-mg tab.

PROBLEM SET	PROBLEM SET ANSWERS

38. Ordered: Amoxicillin 500 mg PO t.i.d.
     Available: Amoxicillin suspension 125 mg/tsp
     Calculate the number of tsp/dose.

38. 4 tsp/dose

39. Ordered: Nicotrol 15 mg/d for 12 wk
     Available: Nicotine Transdermal System 5 mg/d patch
     Calculate the number of patch/d and patches in 12 wk.

39. 3 patch/d
     252 patches/12 wk

40. Ordered: Podophyllum resin 10% in benzoin top for 6 hr; then wash
     with soap and water q.d. for 1 wk
     Available: Podophyllum resin 10% in benzoin
     Convert the dosage to mg/ml.

40. 100 mg/ml

41. Ordered: Ferrous sulfate 10 gr PO b.i.d.
     Available: Ferrous sulfate 300-mg tab
     Calculate the number of tab/dose.

41. 2 tab/dose

PROBLEM SET	PROBLEM SET ANSWERS

42.   Ordered: Atarax 25 mg PO q.i.d. p.r.n.
      Available: Hydroxyzine syrup 10 mg/tsp
      Calculate the number of tsp/dose.

42.   2½ tsp/dose

43.   Ordered: Dicloxacillin 50 mg/kg/d PO q.i.d.
      Available: Dicloxacillin sodium 62.5 mg/5 ml suspension
      Calculate the number of tsp/dose for a patient who weighs 87 lb.

43.   7.9 tsp or 8 tsp/dose

CALCULATIONS FOR ADMINISTRATION OF INTRADERMAL MEDICATIONS AND SKIN TESTS

To place a dose of medication in the dermis layer (the skin) above the subcutaneous tissue (the fat), intradermal medications are given at a 10- to 15-degree angle. The dosage is administered with a large-gauge (small-bore) needle, with its bevel facing up, for comfort and confinement within the dermis layer. The small-bore needle makes a minuscule puncture, that results in minimal postinjection leakage of the medication.

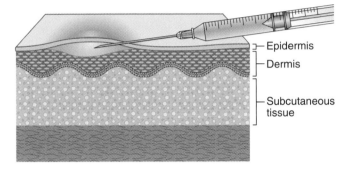

Figure 5–1 *Intradermal placement of a needle at a 10- to 15-degree angle. (From Leahy JM, Nutz P, Administering medications. In Leahy JM, Kizilay PB, eds:* Foundations of Nursing Practice: A Nursing Process Approach. *Philadelphia, WB Saunders, 1998, p. 487 with permission.)*

Typically, you will find that needle gauges range from 16 to 30 G in whole-number increments and in various lengths. For intradermal injection, unless otherwise specified in the order, use a short (⅜ to ½ inch) needle of either 25 or 26 G.

After you finish verifying the provider's orders, follow this procedure to administer intradermal or intracutaneous injections (Fig. 5–2):

The terms *intradermal* and *intracutaneous* are used synonymously for injections close to the surface of the skin and between the layers of the dermis.

1. Choose and prepare the site for injection with an alcohol swab.
2. Allow the alcohol to evaporate from the surface of the skin prior to injection.
3. Hold the syringe parallel to the skin with the tip of the needle barely touching the skin.
4. Stretch the skin away from the tip of the needle and release the skin.
5. Allow the elastic recoil motion of the skin to place the bevel of the needle intradermally.
6. Adjust the needle if necessary.
7. Inject the dosage.
8. Discard the syringe and the needle by placing them in a sharps container (do not recap the needle prior to discarding).

The following are examples of dosage calculations for administration of intradermal medications.

The tuberculin unit (TU) is the standard US unit of measurement for the Siebert-purified protein derivative of tuberculin (PPD). 0.1 ml = 5 TU.

E X A M P L E   1

Ordered: Mantoux tuberculin 5 TU ID now
Available: Tubersol (tuberculin purified protein derivative) 1-ml vial
Calculate the ml/dose (5 TU/0.1 ml).
Pertinent information provided: 5 TU/dose; 5 TU/0.1 ml
Unit equivalency conversion: None needed
Desired unit: ml/dose

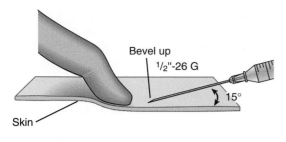

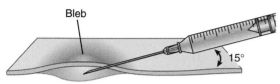

Figure 5–2 *Procedure for administration of intradermal medication.*

Bevel up
¹/₂"-26 G

15°

Skin

1. Pull skin to stretch
2. Place tip of needle to skin
3. Release skin
4. Recoil motion automatically; place needle in position
5. Inject dose

Bleb

15°

CORRECT setup:

$$\frac{5 \; \cancel{TU}}{dose} \times \frac{0.1 \; ml}{5 \; \cancel{TU}} = 0.1 \; ml/dose$$

Ordered × Available =   Answer
  (O)   ×   (A)   =   Ans

 O × A = Ans

E X A M P L E   2

Ordered: Mantoux tuberculin 0.1 ml ID now
Available: Tubersol (tuberculin purified protein derivative) 1-ml vial
Calculate the number of dose/vial.
  Pertinent information provided: 0.1 ml/dose; 1 ml/vial
  Unit equivalency conversion: None needed
  Desired unit: dose/vial

CORRECT setup:

$$\frac{dose}{0.1 \; \cancel{ml}} \times \frac{1 \; \cancel{ml}}{vial} = 10 \; doses/vial$$

   O   ×   A   =   Ans

 The injection site for the Mantoux test is the upper third of the inner fore-arm. Standardizing the location enhances the accuracy of the test read-ing.

E X A M P L E   3

Ordered: PPD tine test
Available: PPD (tuberculin purified protein derivative) tine test
How will you administer this order?
   Cleanse the skin with an alcohol swab and expose the four antigen-coated tines by removing the cap. Press the tines firmly into the skin and hold them in place for at least 1 second. Remove the tines from the skin and dispose of the device by placing it in the sharps container.
   A positive test result for either the Mantoux or the tine test is deter-mined at 48 to 72 hr by the size of the induration measured in millimeters.

 The PPD tine test is a multipuncture, disposable, intradermal test device for administering a tuber-culin test.

 Redness (erythema) with-out firm, raised tissue (induration) is not a posi-tive test.

E X A M P L E   4

Ordered: Cellular hypersensitivity test
Available: Multitest carbohydrate metabolism index (CMI) preloaded sin-gle units

 A multitest unit consists of a plastic applicator tip preloaded (coated) with seven delayed-hypersensi-tivity skin-test antigens.

To prevent the patient from jerking, inform the patient of impending prickling sensations.

 To administer, gently rotate the vial to evenly distribute the particles. Draw 0.1 ml into the tuberculin syringe, and place the dose intradermally. The skin response to the antigen is evaluated in 48 to 72 hr for induration.

 O × A = Ans

 The abbreviations SC and SQ are both used to indicate subcutaneous.

How will you carry out this order?

Before applying, cleanse the area to be injected with an alcohol swab and press the plastic applicator firmly into the skin. The patient's delayed hypersensitivity (allergic) reaction to the antigens of tetanus toxoid, diphtheria toxoid, *Streptococcus,* Old Tuberculin, *Candida, Trichophyton,* and *Proteus* can be assessed in approximately 10 min. The severity of the patient's allergic response is based on the area of redness (erythema) and raised, firm tissue at the test site (induration).

E X A M P L E   5

Ordered: Coccidioidomycosis test ID now
Available: Coccidioidomycosis purified protein antigen 0.1 ml/dose in 1-ml vial
Calculate the number of dose/vial.
   Pertinent information provided: 0.1 ml/dose; 1 ml/vial
   Unit equivalency conversion: None needed
   Desired unit: dose/vial

CORRECT setup:

$$\frac{\text{dose}}{0.1 \text{ ml}} \times \frac{1 \text{ ml}}{\text{vial}} = 10 \text{ doses/vial}$$

CALCULATIONS FOR ADMINISTRATION OF SUBCUTANEOUS MEDICATIONS

Subcutaneous (SC) injections are given at a 45- to 90-degree angle, depending on the length of the needle used and the depth of the subcutaneous tissue. If you use a fairly short needle (that is, ½ to ⅝ inch) on an adult who has a good amount of adipose tissue, you can insert the needle at a 90-degree angle. If you do not have the luxury of choosing the needle length, you will have to either adjust the angle of needle entry or pinch enough of the subcutaneous tissue to administer the dosage.

After you have verified the medication ordered with the provider, you can use this procedure to administer an SC injection.

Figure 5–3 *Needle entering at a 45- to 90-degree angle and reaching the subcutaneous layer. (Modified from Leahy JM, Nutz P, Administering medications. In Leahy JM, Kizilay PB, eds:* Foundations of Nursing Practice: A Nursing Process Approach. *Philadelphia, WB Saunders, 1998, p. 474, with permission.)*

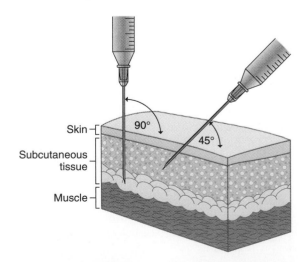

1. Choose the site and prepare it for injection by cleansing it with an alcohol swab.
2. Allow the alcohol to evaporate from the surface of the skin prior to injection.
3. Stabilize the skin for injection by spreading it or pinching a large amount of subcutaneous tissue with your thumb and fourth finger.
4. Place the needle at a 45- or 90-degree angle in the middle of the chosen subcutaneous tissue site.
5. Steady the tip of the syringe next to the skin with your second and third fingers.
6. Aspirate by pulling the plunger with your injecting hand (with heparin, do not aspirate).
7. Inject the contents of the syringe.
8. Pull the needle out gently with a swift and steady motion.
9. Apply gentle pressure over the injection site for several seconds.
10. Do not rub.
11. Dispose of the used syringe and needle in a sharps container.

Insulin Injection

Insulin syringes are available in sizes of 30 U, 50 U, and 100 U. Use the syringe size that is accurately calibrated for you to measure precisely the volume ordered. For example, if you need to draw up 15 U of Humulin, the 30-U syringe will allow you the greatest precision, whereas the 100-U syringe will leave you guessing about the correct calibration mark to measure 15 U. In general, avoid large-volume discrepancies between the volume and the syringe size, for example, don't use a 100-U syringe to measure 3 U.

 Use a syringe that is clearly calibrated to measure the ordered volume.

 Inject insulin and heparin at a 90-degree angle.

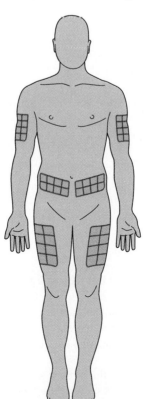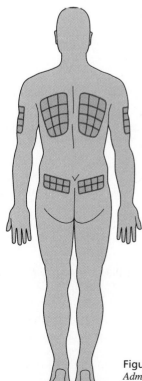

Figure 5–4 *Insulin injection sites. (Modified from Leahy JM, Nutz P, Administering medications. In Leahy JM, Kizilay PB, eds: Foundations of Nursing Practice: A Nursing Process Approach. Philadelphia, WB Saunders, 1998, p. 474, with permission.)*

The abdomen is the preferred site for insulin injections.

Humulin N is also called NPH.

To mix two types of insulin in a single syringe for injection, always draw in the regular (clear) insulin first to avoid contaminating it with the long-acting (cloudy) insulin.

The American Diabetic Association (ADA) recommends using the abdomen as the site for insulin injections. Other less preferred sites are the thighs and the upper arms.

The following are examples of dosage calculations for SC administration.

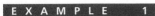

Ordered: Humulin R 10 U mixed with Humulin N 30 U SQ
Available: Humulin R 100 U/ml, 10 ml/vial; Humulin N 100 U/ml, 10 ml/vial

How will you administer this order?

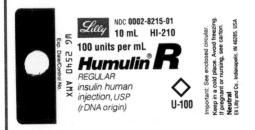

Pertinent information provided: 10 U (R)/dose; 30 U (N)/dose; (R)/100 U ml; 100 U (N)/ml
Unit equivalency conversion: None needed

To administer:

- Cleanse the rubber stoppers of both the insulin R and the insulin N vials with alcohol swabs.
- Obtain an insulin syringe that has a capacity closest to 30 U of insulin (50-U syringe).
- Draw the plunger back to the 30-U mark, inject 30 U of air into the N vial, and remove the syringe.
- Draw the plunger back to the 10-U mark and inject 10 U of air into the R vial.
- Draw in 10 U of insulin R and remove the syringe.
- Insert the needle into the N vial, tilt the vial upside down, and draw up 30 U of N insulin into the syringe.
- Mix the contents of the syringe together by gently rocking the syringe backward and forward.
- Ask another nurse to double-check the dosage order and the amount you have drawn prior to administering the insulin dose to the patient.
- Administer the insulin subcutaneously to a site recommended by the American Diabetic Association.
- Carry out the assessment and evaluation as outlined in the patient's care plan.

If you do not have an insulin syringe, you can use a 1-ml (cc) syringe (30-G, ½-inch needle) to draw up 0.1 ml of Humulin R and then 0.3 ml of Humulin N for this order.

$$\frac{10 \text{ U}}{\text{dose}} \times \frac{\text{ml}}{100 \text{ U (R)}}$$
$$= 0.1 \text{ ml/dose}$$

$$\frac{30 \text{ U}}{\text{dose}} \times \frac{\text{ml}}{100 \text{ U (N)}}$$
$$= 0.3 \text{ ml/dose}$$

Assess the patient after each administration for signs of efficacy and/or signs and symptoms of adverse reactions.

E X A M P L E   2

Ordered: Humulin 70/30 5 U SQ q AM and q PM
Available: Humulin 70/30 100 U/ml in 10-ml vial
How will you administer this order?

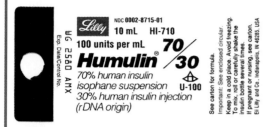

Pertinent information provided: 5 U/dose; 100 U/ml
Unit equivalency conversion: None needed
Desired unit: U/dose
To administer:

- Use a small-volume, 30-U insulin syringe to administer this order.
- Draw 5 U of Humulin 70/30 into the insulin syringe.
- Double-check the dosage with another nurse.
- Administer the dosage after completing the procedure described previously for SC administration.
- Assess and evaluate the patient after dosage administration.

E X A M P L E   3

Ordered: Humulin L 45 U SQ q AM
Available: Humulin Lente 100 U/ml in 10-ml vial
How will you administer this order?

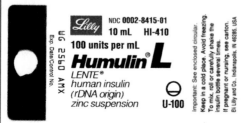

Pertinent information provided: 45 U/dose; 100 U/ml
Unit equivalency conversion: None needed
Desired unit: U/dose

CORRECT setup: None needed

- Draw 45 U of Humulin Lente into a 50-U insulin syringe.
- Double-check the dosage with another nurse.
- Administer the dosage as ordered.
- Do not forget the nursing process.

Humulin 70/30 is a ready-mixed insulin consisting of 70% NPH and 30% R.

For accuracy and precision, use the insulin syringe size that is closest to the order.

Double-check all insulin dosages with another nurse prior to administration.

A patient assessment, a nursing diagnosis, and an evaluation of treatment plan are integral parts of dosage administration.

Standing orders for insulin are given on a sliding-scale basis to allow the adjustment of the dose based on the patient's blood glucose level.

zations, such as measles-mumps-rubella and chickenpox, are given subcutaneously.

Colony-stimulating factors, such as Neupogen, are immune boosters given to increase the number of white blood cells of a patient.

ml/dose = ml/d because the patient is receiving 1 dose/d.

A × O × U × BW = Ans

You may be asked to draw up medication for the provider to administer to the patient.

Lidocaine comes with or without epinephrine. Check the label to make sure you have the correct medication.

You will have a difficult time inserting a 29-G needle through the rubber stopper without bending it.

Use a 26-G, ½-inch needle to inject epinephrine and Sus-Phrine subcutaneously.

A × O × O = Ans

This is a typical example of a dosage based on body weight or body surface area.

EXAMPLE 1

Ordered: Neupogen 2 μg/kg/d SQ until an absolute neutrophil count of 500–1000
Available: Filgrastim 300 μg/ml vial
The patient weighs 95 lb. Calculate the number of ml/dose.
  Pertinent information provided: 2 μg/kg/d; 300 μg/ml; 95 lb
  Unit equivalency conversion: 2.2 lb/kg
  Desired unit: ml/dose (ml/d)

CORRECT setup:

$$\frac{ml}{300\ \mu g} \times \frac{2\ \mu g}{kg \cdot d} \times \frac{kg}{2.2\ lb} \times 95\ lb = 0.288 = 0.29\ ml/dose$$

EXAMPLE 2

Ordered: Xylocaine 10 mg/ml (1%), without epinephrine 3 ml, in a 29-G, 2-inch needle syringe for local anesthetic administration by the provider
Available: Lidocaine HCl, without epinephrine, 10 mg/ml (1%) in 30-ml multiple-dose vial
How will you draw this order?

1. Cleanse the rubber top with an alcohol swab.
2. Use a 3-ml syringe with a 20- or 22-G needle to inject 3 ml of air into the vial.
3. Draw 3 ml of lidocaine into the syringe.
4. Remove the 22-G needle and replace it with a 29-G, 2-inch needle.

EXAMPLE 3

Ordered: Sus-Phrine 25 mg/ml 0.1 ml SQ now
Available: Sus-Phrine (epinephrine) 50 mg/ml, 1-ml vial
Calculate the number of ml/dose.
  Pertinent information provided: 25 mg/ml; 0.1 ml/dose; 50 mg/ml
  Unit equivalency conversion: None needed
  Desired unit: ml/dose

CORRECT setup:

$$\frac{ml}{50\ mg} \times \frac{25\ mg}{ml} \times \frac{0.1\ ml}{dose} = 0.05\ ml/dose$$

EXAMPLE 4

Ordered: Epinephrine 0.01 mg/kg (maximum 0.3 ml) SQ q15–20min p.r.n. for anaphylaxis
Available: Epinephrine 1 mg/ml ampule
Calculate the number of ml/dose for your patient, who weighs 135 lb.

Pertinent information provided: 0.01 mg/kg/dose; 135 lb; maximum 0.3 ml/dose; 1 mg/ml

Unit equivalency conversion: 2.2 lb/kg

Desired unit: ml/dose

CORRECT setup:

$$\frac{1 \text{ ml}}{1 \text{ mg}} \times \frac{0.1 \text{ mg}}{\text{kg} \cdot \text{dose}} \times \frac{\text{kg}}{2.2 \text{ lb}} \times 135 \text{ lb} = 0.6 \text{ ml/dose}$$

Answer: 0.3 ml/dose, because the maximum allowable dose is 0.3 ml/dose

You can set up the problem for unit cancellation, starting with the body weight (BW). The rest will fall into place, that is,

$$135 \text{ lb} \times \frac{\text{kg}}{2.2 \text{ lb}} \times \frac{0.01 \text{ mg}}{\text{kg} \cdot \text{dose}}$$
$$\times \frac{1 \text{ ml}}{1 \text{ mg}} = 0.6 \text{ ml/dose}$$

BW × U × O × A = Ans

As long as all the unwanted units cancel, the position of the conversion factor does not affect the outcome.

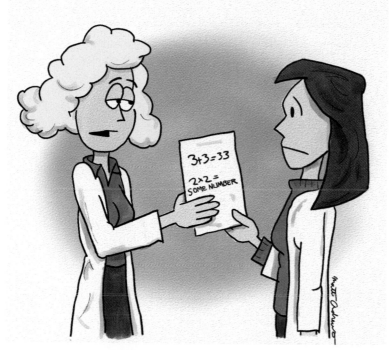

"CHRIS, YOUR SOLUTION TO THIS MEDICATION CALCULATION PROBLEM IS FULL OF CREATIVITY AND IMAGINATION.... WHAT IS MISSING IS LOGIC!"

E X A M P L E   5

Ordered: Dilaudid 0.03 mg/kg SQ q4h

Available: Hydromorphone 1 mg and a 2-mg prefilled Tubex cartridge injection system

Your patient weighs 220 lb. Which cartridge will you choose to administer this order?

Pertinent information provided: 0.03 mg/kg/dose; 220 lb; cartridges: 1 mg/dose; 2 mg/dose

Unit equivalency conversion: 2.2 lb/kg

Desired unit: ml/dose

CORRECT setup:

$$220 \text{ lb} \times \frac{\text{kg}}{2.2 \text{ lb}} \times \frac{0.03 \text{ mg}}{\text{kg} \cdot \text{dose}} = 3 \text{ mg/dose}$$

To avoid injecting the patient twice for this order, you can draw medication out of the prefilled Tubex cartridges as follows:

- Gently remove the needle (with cap in place) from the syringe to expose the rubber cap.
- Use an appropriate syringe and needle to draw the medication out of the Tubex cartridge and through the rubber top.
- Administer the dosage in a single injection.

BW × U × O = Ans

Dilaudid is available in a 4-mg Tubex. With the 4-mg Tubex, you can draw and administer the medication as above.

Answer: Choose one 1-mg and one 2-mg prefilled Tubex cartridges.

The administration, storage, and disposal of medications that are classified as controlled substances must be carried out in strict accordance with established regulatory protocols.

CALCULATIONS FOR ADMINISTRATION OF INTRAMUSCULAR MEDICATIONS

Individuals with a large amount of subcutaneous tissue may require a relatively long needle for the medication to reach the musculature. The choice of the gauge and the length of the needle would depend on the quantity and type of the medication ordered for administration. For example, viscous medications require large-bore needles. Above all, always choose syringes that are calibrated to measure the ordered volume.

Intramuscular injections are given at a 90-degree angle. Additionally, medications that need to be administered into a "deep" intramuscular layer should be given at the gluteal site. The following is a guideline on the maximum volume injectable at the arm, gluteal, and thigh sites for adult and pediatric patients (Pinnell 1996). You will need to adjust these volumes, depending on the physique of your patient, for example, thin versus obese; emaciated from a disease state; bed-bound patients with gross muscular atrophy.

You will notice that the volumes provided under the guideline are further divided in the pediatric population according to age groups. Again, this is

Figure 5–5 *Needle entering at a 90-degree angle and reaching the muscle layer. (Modified from Leahy JM, Nutz P, Administering medications. In Leahy JM, Kizilay PB, eds:* Foundations of Nursing Practice: A Nursing Process Approach. *Philadelphia, WB Saunders, 1998, p. 470 with permission.)*

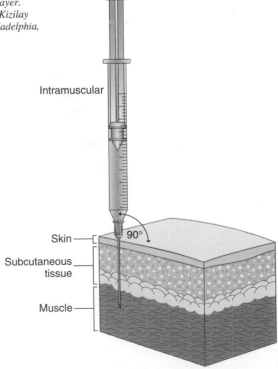

only a guideline. For example, you will not use the gluteal sites (dorsal or ventral) until the child has been actively walking for at least a year. It takes about a year for these muscles to develop adequately for safe administration of intramuscular (IM) injections.

Injection Sites	Landmarks	Maximum Injectable Volumes by Age Group
Deltoid (take care to inject away from the radial nerve)	Acromion, Deltoid muscle, Injection site, Scapula, Deep brachial artery, Radial nerve, Humerus, Axilla	Not appropriate, birth–age 2 0.5 ml Ages 2–3 0.5 ml Ages 3–7 Up to 1 ml ages 7 to 16
Ventrogluteal (the preferred of the two gluteal sites)	Iliac crest, Anterior superior iliac spine, Injection site, Femur	Not appropriate, birth–age 2 1 ml Ages 2–3 1.5 ml Ages 3–7 Up to 2 ml Ages 7–16
Dorsogluteal or gluteus maximus (take care to inject away from the sciatic nerve)	Injection site, Iliac crest, Sciatic nerve, Greater trochanter of femur, Gluteal fold	Not appropriate, birth–age 2 1.0 ml Ages 2–3 1.5 ml Ages 3–7 1.5–2 ml Ages 7–16
Vastus lateralis	Sciatic nerve, Injection site, Vastus lateralis muscle, Femoral artery	0.5–1 ml, Age, birth–age 2 1 ml Ages 2–3 1.5 ml Ages 3–7 1.5–2 ml Ages 7–16
Rectus femoris	Sciatic nerve, Rectus femoris muscle, Injection site, Vastus lateralis muscle, Femoral artery	0.5–1 ml, Age, birth–age 2 1 ml Ages 2–3 1.5 ml Ages 3–7 1.5–2 ml Ages 7–16

The figures in this table are from O'Toole MR, ed: Miller-Keane Encyclopedia and Dictionary of Medicine, Nursing, and Allied Health. 6th ed. Philadelphia, WB Saunders, 1997, p. 832, with permission.

The following procedure is used to administer an IM dose of medication:

1. Select the site and prepare the area for administration, for example, deltoid muscle, gluteal muscle.
2. Spread the skin taut with your dominant hand.
3. Using a swift motion, place the needle into the muscular layer.
4. Release the skin.
5. With your free hand, hold the base of the needle to keep the syringe steady.
6. Aspirate the plunger with the other hand.
7. Inject the medication as ordered.
8. Using a swift and uniform motion, remove the needle.
9. Apply gentle pressure over the injection site for several seconds.
10. If bleeding occurs, apply a dry dressing, for example, a BandAid.
11. Dispose of the syringe and the needle by placing them in a sharps container.

The following are examples of dosage calculations for the IM administration of medications and immunizations.

Always aspirate before injecting the ordered immunization dosage.

E X A M P L E   1

Ordered: DPT toxoid 0.5 ml IM now
Available: DPT toxoid suspension in a 5-ml vial
Calculate the number of available dose/vial.
Pertinent information provided: 0.5 ml/dose; 5 ml/vial
Unit equivalency conversion: None needed
Desired unit: dose/vial

CORRECT setup:

$$\frac{dose}{0.5 \ \text{ml}} \times \frac{5 \ \text{ml}}{vial} = 10 \text{ dose/vial}$$

O × A = Answer

E X A M P L E   2

Ordered: Flu-Immune 0.25 ml IM now
Available: Flu-Immune (influenza purified surface antigen) 5-ml vial
Calculate the number of dose/vial.
Pertinent information provided: 0.25 ml/dose; 5 ml/vial
Unit equivalency conversion: None needed
Desired unit: dose/vial

CORRECT setup:

$$\frac{dose}{0.25 \ \text{ml}} \times \frac{5 \ \text{ml}}{vial} = 20 \text{ dose/vial}$$

Flu-Immune 0.25 ml is a pediatric dosage. Adults require 0.5 ml/dose. Administer Flu-Immune into the deltoid muscle. Explain to the patient the possible adverse effects of the immunization and obtain a signed consent prior to the administration of the immunization.

O × A = Ans

HibTITER is given to immunize children 2 to 71 mo of age against *Haemophilus* b disease.

E X A M P L E   3

Ordered: HibTITER 0.5 ml IM now
Available: HibTITER (*Haemophilus* b conjugate vaccine) 5-ml vial
Calculate the number of dose/vial.

Pertinent information provided: 0.5 ml/dose; 5 ml/vial
Unit equivalency conversion: None needed
Desired unit: dose/vial

CORRECT setup:

$$\frac{\text{dose}}{0.5 \text{ ml}} \times \frac{5 \text{ ml}}{\text{vial}} = 10 \text{ dose/vial}$$

 O × A = Ans

E X A M P L E   4

Ordered: Hep-B-Gammagee 0.5 ml IM now
Available: Hep-B-Gammagee (hepatitis B immune globulin) 5-ml vial
Calculate the number of dose/vial.
Pertinent information provided: 0.5 ml/dose; 5 ml/vial
Unit equivalency conversion: None needed
Desired unit: dose/vial

Hepatitis B vaccine (Recombivax HB) immunization requires three shots given at 0, 1, and 6 mo intervals.

CORRECT setup:

$$\frac{\text{dose}}{0.5 \text{ ml}} \times \frac{5 \text{ ml}}{\text{vial}} = 10 \text{ dose/vial}$$

 O × A = Ans

E X A M P L E   5

Ordered: Ampicillin sodium 500 mg IM single dose now
Available: Sterile ampicillin sodium 1 gm reconstituted to 4 ml

M I N I   Q U I Z

What site is preferred for administering this medication, and why?

Answer: The gluteal site, because IM antibiotic injections require a large muscle mass with adequate circulation. Also, the dose is quite large.

Calculate the number of ml necessary for this order.

NDC 0015-7404-20
NSN 6505-00-993-3518
EQUIVALENT TO
1 gram AMPICILLIN
STERILE AMPICILLIN SODIUM, USP
For IM or IV Use
CAUTION: Federal law prohibits dispensing without prescription.
APOTHECON

For IM use, add 3.5 mL diluent (read accompanying circular). Resulting solution contains 250 mg ampicillin per mL.
Use solution within 1 hour.
This vial contains ampicillin sodium equivalent to 1 gram ampicillin.
Usual Dosage: Adults—250 to 500 mg IM q 6h.
READ ACCOMPANYING CIRCULAR for detailed indications, IM or IV dosage and precautions.
APOTHECON®
A Bristol-Myers Squibb Company
Princeton, NJ 08540 USA

740420DRL-2

Cont:
Exp. Date:

Pertinent information provided: 500 mg/dose; 1 gm/4 ml
Unit equivalency conversion: None needed
Desired unit: ml/dose

CORRECT setup:

$$\frac{4 \text{ ml}}{1 \text{ gm}} \times \frac{1 \text{ gm}}{1000 \text{ mg}} \times \frac{500 \text{ mg}}{\text{dose}} = 2 \text{ ml/dose}$$

 A × O = Ans

To decrease pain at the injection site, it is recommended that Rocephin be diluted with 1% lidocaine solution (without epinephrine), for example, inject 0.9 ml of 1% lidocaine into a 250-mg vial to get 250 mg/ml Rocephin.

Look for the instructions on the vial to reconstitute the powdered medication.

A × O × U = Ans

The largest IM injection volume considered safe is 3 ml.

A × O × U = Ans

Gauges of 27 and higher are too soft to penetrate rubber stoppers. Gauges of 22 and higher are too small to draw in viscous (thick) medications.

Answer: Gently but firmly push the needle (with the cap in place) into the Tubex syringe until you feel a "pop." Connect the Tubex injector to the cartridge. Push out the excess air before you inject.

E X A M P L E   6

Ordered: Rocephin 1 gm IM now
Available: Rocephin (ceftriaxone sodium) 250 mg/ml vial
Calculate the number of ml/dose. How would you administer this order?
Pertinent information provided: 1 gm/dose; 250 mg/ml
Unit equivalency conversion: 1000 mg/gm
Desired unit: ml/dose

CORRECT setup:

$$\frac{ml}{250\ \cancel{mg}} \times \frac{1\ \cancel{gm}}{dose} \times \frac{1000\ \cancel{mg}}{\cancel{gm}} = 4\ ml/dose$$

Administer this order in two separate injections of 2 ml, because 4 ml of Rocephin is too large a volume to administer in a single injection at any of the intramuscular sites.

E X A M P L E   7

Ordered: Vitamin B_{12} 100 µg IM now
Available: Cyanocobalamin injection 1 mg/ml 30-ml vial
Calculate the number of ml/dose.
Pertinent information provided: 100 µg/dose; 1 mg/ml
Unit equivalency conversion: 1000 µg/mg
Desired unit: ml/dose

CORRECT setup:

$$\frac{ml}{1\ \cancel{mg}} \times \frac{100\ \cancel{\mu g}}{dose} \times \frac{1\ \cancel{mg}}{1000\ \cancel{\mu g}} = 0.1\ ml/dose$$

- If you use a different needle to draw the medication into the syringe, remember to pull the plunger away from the needle.
- Change to the needle you will be using to inject the medication and gently push up a small amount of medication to displace the air in the new needle.
- Administer the medication as ordered.

E X A M P L E   8

Ordered: Toradol 60 mg IM now
Available: Ketorolac tromethamine 60 mg/ml Tubex cartridge-needle unit

M I N I   Q U I Z

How would you administer this order?

Calculate the number of ml/dose.
Pertinent information provided: 60 mg/dose; 60 mg/ml
Unit equivalency conversion: None needed
Desired unit: ml/dose

CORRECT setup:

$$\frac{\text{ml}}{60 \text{ mg}} \times \frac{60 \text{ mg}}{\text{dose}} = 1 \text{ ml/dose}$$

A × O = Ans

E X A M P L E   9

Ordered: Depo-Provera 150 mg IM q3mo
Available: Medroxyprogesterone acetate 150 mg/ml aqueous suspension vial
Calculate the number of ml/dose.
    Pertinent information provided: 150 mg/dose; 150 mg/ml
    Unit equivalency conversion: None needed
    Desired unit: ml/dose

Know the generic, chemical, and trade names of medications.

Obtain a signature on an informed consent form prior to administration of contraceptive agents. Give by deep IM injection into the gluteal or deltoid muscle.

CORRECT setup:

$$\frac{\text{ml}}{150 \text{ mg}} \times \frac{150 \text{ mg}}{\text{dose}} = 1 \text{ ml/dose}$$

A × O = Ans

E X A M P L E   1 0

Ordered: Morphine sulfate ¼ gr
Available: Morphine sulfate 15 mg/ml vial
Calculate the number of ml/dose.

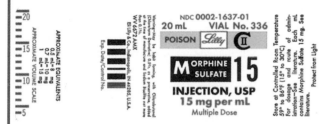

Follow the protocols set by each institution regarding storage, administration, and disposal of controlled substances.

    Pertinent information provided: ¼ gr/dose; 15 mg/ml
    Unit equivalency conversion: 60 mg/gr
    Desired unit: ml/dose

Double-check the amount of the dosage with another nurse prior to administration of controlled substances.

CORRECT setup:

$$\frac{\text{ml}}{15 \text{ mg}} \times \frac{1 \text{ gr}}{4 \text{ dose}} \times \frac{60 \text{ mg}}{\text{gr}} = 1 \text{ ml/dose}$$

A × O × U = Ans

E X A M P L E   1 1

Ordered: Solganal 20 mg IM now
Available: Aurothioglucose 5% (50 mg/ml) 10-ml vial
Calculate the number of ml/dose.
    Pertinent information provided: 20 mg/dose; 50 mg/ml
    Unit equivalency conversion: None needed
    Desired unit: ml/dose

Solganal is extremely viscous and must be drawn up with a large-bore needle (<20 G).

CORRECT setup:

$$\frac{\text{ml}}{50 \text{ mg}} \times \frac{20 \text{ mg}}{\text{dose}} = 0.4 \text{ ml/dose}$$

A × O = Ans

To administer:

- Rotate the vial vigorously.
- Use a large-bore needle (18 G) to draw up the medication.
- For the patient's comfort, use a smaller bore needle (22 G) to inject.
- Use the Z-tract method to inject by stretching the skin away before placement of the needle.
- Slowly remove the needle and apply firm pressure. If necessary, place a Band-Aid over the site.

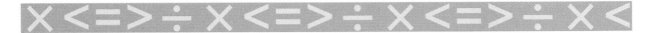

Chapter Summary

We have demonstrated that most intradermal, SC, and IM dosage calculations can be accomplished by multiplying the conversion factors of the available dosages and the ordered dosages. If you are having difficulty in conceptualizing parenteral dosage calculations using dimensional analysis, you will need to review Chapter 3. The following is a list of reminders:

✔ Remember to read the problem carefully.
✔ Ask yourself if you have a clear understanding of what the problem is asking you to do.
✔ Make sure you apply the necessary unit equivalence conversion factor(s) in your setup.
✔ Remember that to cancel, you must have the same unit in the numerator and the denominator.
✔ Check that the math is done accurately.

PROBLEM SET	PROBLEM SET ANSWERS
1. Ordered: Morphine sulfate 1/60 gr IM now Available: Morphine sulfate 1 mg/ml Calculate number of ml/dose.	1. 1 ml/dose
2. Ordered: Demerol 1 mg/kg IM q4hr Available: Meperidine 25 mg/ml Carpuject cartridge-needle Calculate the number of ml/dose for a patient who weighs 186 lb.	2. 3.38 = 3.4 ml/dose

PROBLEM SET	PROBLEM SET ANSWERS

3. Ordered: Morphine sulfate 8 mg IM q4hr.
Available: Morphine sulfate 15 mg/ml
Calculate the number of ml/dose.

3. 0.53 ml/dose

4. Ordered: Humulin N 30 U SQ now
Available: NPH 100 U/ml
Calculate the number of U/dose.

4. 30 U/dose

5. Ordered: Heparin 20,000 U SQ stat
Available: Heparin 10,000 U/ml 10-ml vial
Calculate the number of ml/dose.

5. 2 ml/dose

6. Ordered: Sus-Phrine 1:200 0.15 ml SQ stat
Available: Sus-Phrine (epinephrine) 1:200 5-ml vial
Calculate the number of ml/dose.

6. 0.15 ml

7. Ordered: Roferon-A 36,000,000 IU IM q.d.
Available: Roferon-A (interferon alpha-2a [recombinant])
9,000,000 IU/ml vial
Calculate the number of ml/dose.

7. 4 ml/dose

   Divide dose into two injections before administering.

CALCULATIONS FOR ADMINISTRATION OF PERIPHERAL SOLUTIONS

Intravenous solutions are used to replace or maintain fluid and/or electrolytes. There are many different kinds of IV fluids with varying types and concentrations of electrolytes. The most common ones that you will see are 0.9% sodium chloride (normal saline solution), and 5% dextrose solution (D_5W solution). In the United States, most IV fluids are packaged in calibrated plastic bags or glass bottles, and the respective contents are clearly labeled on the package.

The provider initiates the order for an IV fluid, but the nurse is responsible for administering the fluid as ordered. If a fluid volume infusion pump unit is available, the rate of infusion can be programmed into the pump, for example 125 ml/hr, 30 ml/hr; otherwise, the nurse must determine the drip rate in drops per minute to administer the ordered IV fluid accurately.

 It is prudent to check the drip rate delivered by the volume infusion pump to make sure it is in good working order.

Even when one uses a volume infusion pump, it is best not to be lulled into trusting its accuracy when administering intravenous fluids and medications. Machines can break or malfunction. It is up to the nurse to calculate the flow rate or drip rate and to double-check the accuracy of the volume infusion pump. How else is the nurse to be sure that the volume infusion pump is operating properly?

To administer an IV fluid to your patient, use the following procedure:

1. Apply the three checks and the five rights in the selection of IV fluids ordered.
2. Remove the tab or cap that seals the outflow access on the bag or bottle.
3. Select a primary line that has an appropriate drip chamber, that is, micro- or macrodrop, with a sufficient length of tubing and number of ports.
4. Close the clamp. This will prevent air from entering the line during priming.
5. Connect the drip chamber to your IV bag or bottle by placing the spike into the IV bag or bottle's outflow access.
6. Open the clamp to prime the line, allowing the fluid to displace the air in the tubing by running the fluid into the drip chamber and the attached tubing.
7. Close the clamp when the tubing is filled.
8. Review the three checks and the five rights before you attach the connector at the end of the tubing to your patient's IV catheter.
9. Open the clamp carefully to allow the IV fluid to flow at the ordered drip rate.

 Drop size depends on the manufacturer of the administration set.

Most well-equipped hospitals have IV volume infusion pumps for administration of fluids and medication. However, depending on geographic locale, health institutions vary in available resources and supportive technology in patient care. Therefore, you will need to know how to calculate drip rates. The volume infusion pump allows you to enter flow-rate data as ordered, for example, volume (ml), time (min, hr).

Drip rates are calculated in drops per minute. Drop factors can be micro- or macrodrop. Macrodrop factors range from 10 drops/ml to 20 drops/ml, depending on the manufacturer. The microdrop factor is uniformly set at 60 μgtt/ml.

The following are examples of IV fluid drip-rate calculations.

IV drip rate = gtt/min
or μgtt/min
μgtt/ml = 60 μgtt/ml
gtt/ml = 10 to 20 gtt/ml

IV flow rate = ml/hr

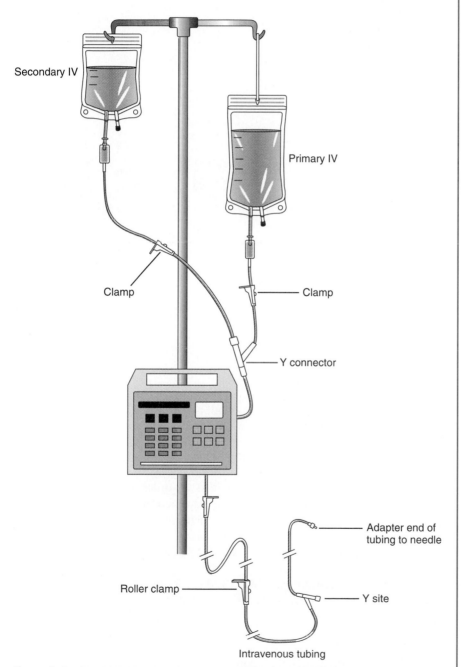

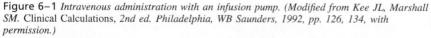

Figure 6–1 *Intravenous administration with an infusion pump. (Modified from Kee JL, Marshall SM. Clinical Calculations, 2nd ed. Philadelphia, WB Saunders, 1992, pp. 126, 134, with permission.)*

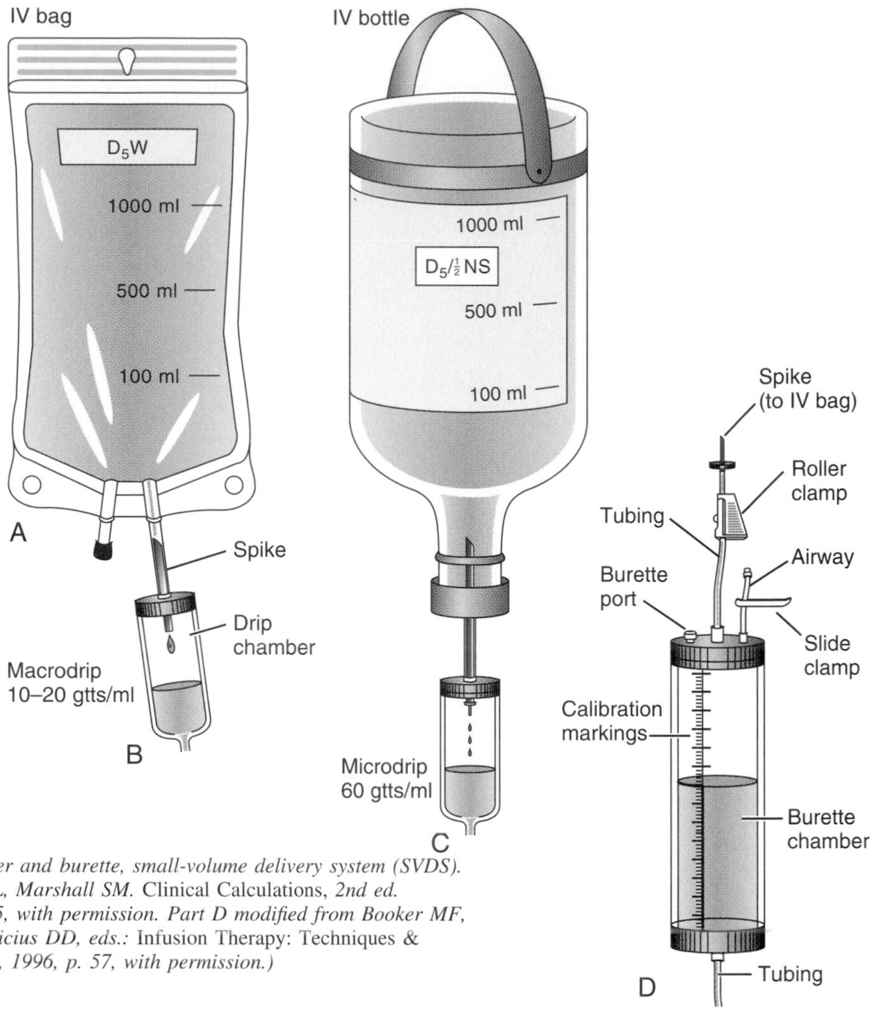

IV bag

D₅W

1000 ml —

500 ml —

100 ml —

A

Spike

Drip chamber

Macrodrip
10–20 gtts/ml

B

IV bottle

1000 ml —

D₅/½ NS

500 ml —

100 ml —

Microdrip
60 gtts/ml

C

Spike
(to IV bag)

Roller clamp

Tubing

Airway

Burette port

Slide clamp

Calibration markings

Burette chamber

Tubing

D

Figure 6–2 *Bag/bottle with drip chamber and burette, small-volume delivery system (SVDS).*
(Parts A, B, and C modified from Kee JL, Marshall SM. Clinical Calculations, *2nd ed.*
Philadelphia, WB Saunders, 1992, p. 125, with permission. Part D modified from Booker MF,
Infusion systems. In Booker MF, Ignatavicius DD, eds.: Infusion Therapy: Techniques &
Medications. *Philadelphia, WB Saunders, 1996, p. 57, with permission.)*

 Ask yourself the following questions: What is the problem asking you to solve? What information is provided? What additional information, such as unit equivalency, is needed? Did you place the desired unit in the orientation that you need? Did all of the unwanted units cancel? Is your arithmetic correct?

 DF = 15 gtt/ml
Ov = 1 L/dose
Ot = 8 hr/dose
DF × U × Ov × Ot × U = Ans

 Round the answer: A drop cannot be split in the drip chamber.

EXAMPLE 1

Ordered: D₅W 1 L q8hr

Calculate the drip rate in gtt/min (15 gtt/ml).

The problem can be interpreted as follows:
You need to administer 1 L of fluid, that is, ordered volume (Ov), D₅W, over an 8-hr period of time, that is, ordered time (Ot). Imagine a bag of 1 L of D₅W attached to a macrodrop drip chamber set to deliver 15 gtt/ml of fluid, that is, the drop factor (DF). The problem is asking you to calculate the number of drops that you will see falling into the drip chamber over a 1-min period of time.

Pertinent information provided: 1 L/dose; 8 hr/dose; 15 gtt/ml (DF)
Unit equivalency conversion: 1000 ml/L; 60 min/hr
Desired unit: gtt/min

CORRECT setup:

$$\frac{15 \text{ gtt}}{\text{ml}} \times \frac{1000 \text{ ml}}{\text{L}} \times \frac{1 \text{ L}}{\text{dose}} \times \frac{\text{dose}}{8 \text{ hr}} \times \frac{1 \text{ hr}}{60 \text{ min}} = 31.25 = 31 \text{ gtt/min}$$

DF   ×   U   × Ov × Ot ×   U   = Ans

EXAMPLE   2

Ordered: NS 500 ml over 1 hr

Calculate the drip rate in gtt/min (20 gtt/ml).

Pertinent information provided: 500 ml/dose; 1 hr/dose; 20 gtt/ml

Unit equivalency conversion: 60 min/hr

Desired unit: gtt/min

CORRECT setup:

$$\frac{20 \text{ gtt}}{\text{ml}} \times \frac{500 \text{ ml}}{\text{dose}} \times \frac{\text{dose}}{1 \text{ hr}} \times \frac{1 \text{ hr}}{60 \text{ min}} = 166.6 = 167 \text{ gtt/min}$$

DF = 20 gtt/ml
Ov = 500 ml/dose
Ot = 1 hr/dose

DF × Ov × Ot × U =
Ans

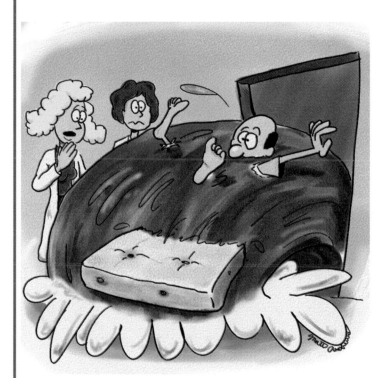

"I'M SURE I CALCULATED MR. SMYTH'S
DRIP RATE CORRECTLY!"

EXAMPLE   3

Ordered: Lactated Ringer's solution 1 L q10hr

Calculate the drip rate in gtt/min (15 gtt/ml).

Pertinent information provided: 1 L/dose; 10 hr/dose; 15 gtt/ml

Unit equivalency conversion: 1000 ml/L; 60 min/hr

Desired unit: gtt/min

CORRECT setup:

$$\frac{15 \text{ gtt}}{\text{ml}} \times \frac{1000 \text{ ml}}{\text{L}} \times \frac{1 \text{ L}}{\text{dose}} \times \frac{\text{dose}}{10 \text{ hr}} \times \frac{1 \text{ hr}}{60 \text{ min}} = 25 \text{ gtt/min}$$

DF = 15 gtt/ml
Ov = 1 L/dose
Ot = 10 hr/dose

DF × U × Ov × Ot ×
U = Ans

DF = 60 μgtt/ml
Ov = 50 ml/dose
Ot = 1 hr/dose

To keep time, count the drops per second by saying, "crocodile," or "tired nurse," for example, one tired nurse, two tired nurses, three tired. . . .

DF × Ov × Ot × U = Ans

It is impossible to count drops with a fast running IV. You will see a stream running through the drip chamber instead of individual drops.

DF = 60 μgtt/ml
Ov = 50 ml/dose
Ot = 20 min/dose

Answer: No. This system is too fast to see the drops clearly at 150 μgtt/min.

DF = 15 gtt/ml
Ov = 1 L/dose
Ot = 2 hr/dose

DF × U × Ov × Ot × U = Ans

EXAMPLE 4

Ordered: D$_5$W 50 ml in 1 hr
Calculate the drip rate in μgtt/min (60 μgtt/ml).
   Pertinent information provided: 50 ml/dose; 1 hr/dose; 60 μgtt/ml
   Unit equivalency conversion: 60 min/hr
   Desired unit: μgtt/min

CORRECT setup:

$$\frac{60\ \mu\text{gtt}}{\text{ml}} \times \frac{50\ \text{ml}}{\text{dose}} \times \frac{\text{dose}}{1\ \text{hr}} \times \frac{1\ \text{hr}}{60\ \text{min}} = 50\ \mu\text{gtt/min}$$

Would you consider using a macrodrop chamber? At this rate, it is a judgment call. Drip rates faster than 60 μgtt/min will require a macrodrop system because you cannot count the drops fast enough for accuracy.

EXAMPLE 5

Ordered: NS 50 ml in 20 min
Calculate the drip rate in μgtt/min (60 μgtt/ml).

MINI QUIZ

Will you use a microdrop system to administer this order?

   Pertinent information provided: 50 ml/dose; 20 min/dose; 60 μgtt/ml
   Unit equivalency conversion: None needed
   Desired unit: μgtt/min

CORRECT setup:

$$\frac{60\ \mu\text{gtt}}{\text{ml}} \times \frac{50\ \text{ml}}{\text{dose}} \times \frac{\text{dose}}{20\ \text{min}} = 150\ \mu\text{gtt/min}$$
$$\quad\ \ \text{DF}\quad \times \quad \text{Ov}\quad \times \quad \text{Ot}\quad = \quad\ \text{Ans}$$

EXAMPLE 6

Ordered: ½ NS 1 L over 2 hr
Calculate the drip rate in gtt/min (15 gtt/ml).
   Pertinent information provided: 1 L/dose; 2 hr/dose; 15 gtt/ml
   Unit equivalency conversion: 1000 ml/L; 60 min/hr
   Desired unit: gtt/min

CORRECT setup:

$$\frac{15\ \text{gtt}}{\text{ml}} \times \frac{1000\ \text{ml}}{\text{L}} \times \frac{1\ \text{L}}{\text{dose}} \times \frac{\text{dose}}{2\ \text{hr}} \times \frac{1\ \text{hr}}{60\ \text{min}} = 125\ \text{gtt/min}$$

EXAMPLE 7

Ordered: D₅W 500 ml over 6 hr
Calculate the flow rate in μgtt/min (60 μgtt/ml).
   Pertinent information provided: 500 ml/dose; 6 hr/dose; 60 μgtt/ml
   Unit equivalency conversion: 60 min/hr
   Desired unit: μgtt/min

CORRECT setup:

$$\frac{60\ \mu gtt}{\cancel{ml}} \times \frac{500\ \cancel{ml}}{\cancel{dose}} \times \frac{\cancel{dose}}{6\ \cancel{hr}} \times \frac{1\ \cancel{hr}}{60\ min} = 83.33 = 83\ \mu gtt/min$$

DF = 60 μgtt/ml
Ov = 500 ml/dose
Ot = 6 hr/dose

DF × Ov × Ot × U = Ans

EXAMPLE 8

Ordered: NS 500 ml over 12 hr
Calculate the drip rate in μgtt/min.
   Pertinent information provided: 500 ml/dose; 12 hr/dose; 60 μgtt/ml
   Unit equivalency conversion: 60 min/hr
   Desired unit: μgtt/min

CORRECT setup:

$$\frac{60\ \mu gtt}{\cancel{ml}} \times \frac{500\ \cancel{ml}}{\cancel{dose}} \times \frac{\cancel{dose}}{12\ \cancel{hr}} \times \frac{1\ \cancel{hr}}{60\ min} = 41.66 = 42\ \mu gtt/min$$

DF = 60 μgtt/ml
Ov = 500 ml/dose
Ot = 12 hr/dose

DF × Ov × Ot × U = Ans

EXAMPLE 9

Ordered: NS 1 L KVO (40 ml/hr)
Calculate the drip rate in gtt/min (15 gtt/ml).
   Pertinent information provided: 40 ml/hr; 15 gtt/ml
   Unit equivalency conversion: 60 min/hr
   Desired unit: gtt/min

CORRECT setup:

$$\frac{15\ gtt}{\cancel{ml}} \times \frac{40\ \cancel{ml}}{\cancel{hr}} \times \frac{1\ \cancel{hr}}{60\ min} = 10\ gtt/min$$

KVO translates to "keep vein open." It requires fluids to be administered at approximately 30 to 40 ml/hr.
DF = 15 gtt/ml
Or = 40 ml/hr

DF × Or × U = Ans

EXAMPLE 10

Ordered: NS 1 L KVO (40 ml/hr)
Calculate the drip rate in μgtt/min.
   Pertinent information provided: 40 ml/hr; 60 μgtt/ml
   Unit equivalency conversion: 60 min/hr
   Desired unit: μgtt/min

CORRECT setup:

$$\frac{60\ \mu gtt}{\cancel{ml}} \times \frac{40\ ml}{hr} \times \frac{1\ hr}{60\ min} = 40\ \mu gtt/min$$

DF = 60 μgtt/ml
Or = 30 ml/hr

Notice how the 60 (μgtt) and the 60 (min) cancel each other, leaving you with the 40 (ml). Flow rate = drip rate with the microdrop system.
DF × Or × U = Ans

CALCULATIONS FOR ADMINISTRATION OF PERIPHERAL MEDICATIONS

Intravenous medication dosage orders can be categorized as follows:

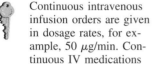

Continuous intravenous infusion orders are given in dosage rates, for example, 50 μg/min. Continuous IV medications are frequently ordered in dose/time unit, for example, mg/min, μg/min.

- Intravenous slow push (IVSP): Medication ordered to be administered slowly into the peripheral venous access through the port closest to the catheter, or directly into a catheter lock.
- Continuous intravenous drip: Medication ordered to be administered continuously over a specified period of time. The orders for continuous IV drip administration of medication are written in amount/time, for example, mg/hr, μg/min, mEq/hr.
- Intravenous piggyback (IVPB): medication ordered to be administered via a secondary system attached to the primary IV fluid administration system. The secondary system must be elevated above the primary system for fluid to flow. Whenever the order lacks a time specification, IVPB medications are administered over 20 to 30 min for 50 ml, and 60 min (1 hr) for 100-ml volumes.

Figure 6–3 *Intravenous administration system for blood transfusion. (From O'Toole MT, ed.: Miller-Keane Encyclopedia and Dictionary of Medicine, Nursing, and Allied Health, 6th ed. Philadelphia, WB Saunders, 1997, p. 1761, with permission.)*

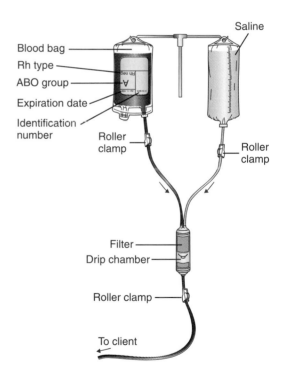

Y-connector blood administration set. Redrawn from Lammon et al., 1995.

Because the medication or blood product is administered directly into the circulatory system, there is absolutely no room for error. Therefore, you need to make sure you understand the order clearly, and you need to go through the three checks and the five rights. Above all, look up all medications that are unfamiliar to you and take a little time to know your patient's health history, for example, the nature of the illness diagnosed, multiple medications, allergies.

You will need to follow the institution's protocol to administer blood or blood products. Here is a basic guideline:

- Obtain identification of the blood product and the recipient.
- Validate the identification with at least two other nurses.
- Check, check, and check again the type and the compatibility between the recipient and the blood product, that is, A, B, O, and Rh.
- Implement the nursing process pertinent to blood and/or blood product administration, for example, adverse reactions.

Without a volume infusion pump, you will need to place the secondary system higher than the primary system.

Administer the IVSP dosage at a rate recommended by the manufacturer of the medication. Frequently, IVPB dosages are ordered to be administered over 30 min. You can safely administer IVPB dosages over 30 min if you do not have access to the manufacturer's guidelines or if you cannot consult a pharmacist.

The following are examples of IVSP, continuous IV, and IVPB dosage calculations. The IVSP and IVPB modes of administration are also called intermittent intravenous infusions.

E X A M P L E   1

Ordered: Premarin 25 mg IVSP stat and repeat in 6 hr p.r.n.
Available: Premarin (conjugated estrogen) 25 mg/vial reconstitute with 5-ml diluent containing 2% benzyl alcohol in sterile water
Calculate the number of vials/dose.
  Pertinent information provided: 25 mg/dose; 25 mg/vial
  Unit equivalency conversion: None needed
  Desired unit: vial/dose

CORRECT setup:

$$\frac{1 \text{ vial}}{25 \text{ mg}} \times \frac{25 \text{ mg}}{\text{dose}} = 1 \text{ vial/dose}$$

Prior to reconstituting the medication, carefully read the directions that are provided on the vial and package inserts.

A × O = Ans

E X A M P L E   2

Ordered: Reglan 5 mg IVSP q6hr
Available: Reglan (metoclopramide monohydrochloride monohydrate) 10 mg/ml
Calculate the number of ml/dose.
  Pertinent information provided: 5 mg/dose; 10 mg/ml
  Unit equivalency conversion: None needed
  Desired unit: ml/dose

CORRECT setup:

$$\frac{\text{ml}}{10 \text{ mg}} \times \frac{5 \text{ mg}}{\text{dose}} = \frac{1}{2} \text{ ml/dose}$$

IVSP dosage problems are solved by using the same setup as the injectable dosages presented in Chapter 5.

A × O = Ans

Always use the volume
in the secondary system
to calculate parenteral
dosages.
DF = 15 gtt/ml
Ov = 100 ml/dose
Ot = 30 min/dose

E X A M P L E   3

Ordered: Cefuroxime sodium 1500 mg IVPB over 30 min
Available: Kefurox 1.5 gm in 100 ml of NS (The pharmacy delivered it
ready to administer.)
Calculate the drip rate in gtt/min (15 gtt/ml).

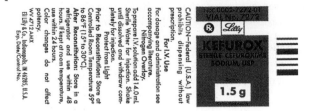

Pertinent information provided: 100 ml/dose; 30 min/dose; 15 gtt/ml
Unit equivalency conversion: None needed
Desired unit: gtt/min

CORRECT setup:

DF × Ov × Ot = Ans

$$\frac{15 \text{ gtt}}{\text{ml}} \times \frac{100 \text{ ml}}{\text{dose}} \times \frac{\text{dose}}{30 \text{ min}} = 50 \text{ gtt/min}$$

E X A M P L E   4

Ordered: Kytril 1 mg IVPB in 50 ml of D_5W over 20 min
Available: Kytril (granisetron HCl) 1 mg/ml in 1-ml vial

DF = 20 gtt/ml
Ov = 50 ml/dose
Ot = 20 min/dose

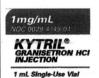

Calculate the drip rate in gtt/min (20 gtt/ml).
Pertinent information provided: 50 ml/dose; 20 min/dose; 20 gtt/ml
Unit equivalency conversion: None needed
Desired unit: gtt/min

DF × Ov × Ot = Ans

CORRECT setup:

$$\frac{20 \text{ gtt}}{\text{ml}} \times \frac{50 \text{ ml}}{\text{dose}} \times \frac{\text{dose}}{20 \text{ min}} = 50 \text{ gtt/min}$$

E X A M P L E   5

Ordered: Sus-Phrine 50 μg/min continuous IV
Available: Sus-Phrine (epinephrine) 5 mg in 500 ml of NS

1. Calculate the drip rate in gtt/min (10 gtt/ml).
2. Calculate the flow rate in ml/hr.

You will need to calcu-
late the flow of a volume
infusion pump in ml/hr.
DF = 10 gtt/ml
A = 5 mg/500 ml
Or = 50 μg/min

Pertinent information provided: 50 μg/min; 5 mg/500 ml; 10 gtt/ml
Unit equivalency conversion: 1000 μg/mg
Desired units: (1) gtt/min (drip rate); (2) ml/hr (flow rate)

CORRECT setup:

1. gtt/min:

$$\frac{10 \text{ gtt}}{\text{ml}} \times \frac{500 \text{ ml}}{5 \text{ mg}} \times \frac{1 \text{ mg}}{1000 \text{ μg}} \times \frac{50 \text{ μg}}{\text{min}} = 50 \text{ gtt/min}$$

DF × A × U × Or =
Ans

2. ml/hr:

$$\frac{500 \text{ ml}}{5 \text{ mg}} \times \frac{1 \text{ mg}}{1000 \text{ μg}} \times \frac{50 \text{ μg}}{\text{min}} \times \frac{60 \text{ min}}{\text{hr}} = 300 \text{ ml/hr}$$

A × U × Or × U = Ans

E X A M P L E   6

Ordered: Morphine sulfate 2 mg/hr IV
Available: Morphine sulfate 100 mg in 250 ml D_5W (dextrose in water)

1. Calculate the drip rate in μgtt/min.
2. Calculate the flow rate in ml/hr.

Pertinent information provided: 2 mg/hr; 100 mg/250 ml; 60 μgtt/ml
Unit equivalency conversion: 60 min/hr
Desired units: (1) μgtt/min (drip rate); (2) ml/hr (flow rate)

DF = 60 μgtt/ml
Or = 2 mg/hr
A = 100 mg/250 ml

CORRECT setup:

1. μgtt/min:

$$\frac{60 \text{ μgtt}}{\text{ml}} \times \frac{250 \text{ ml}}{100 \text{ mg}} \times \frac{2 \text{ mg}}{\text{hr}} \times \frac{\text{hr}}{60 \text{ min}} = 5 \text{ μgtt/min}$$

Remember the 60 (μgtt) and the 60 (min) cancel each other. So if you want, you can leave them out of your setup.

2. ml/hr:

$$\frac{250 \text{ ml}}{100 \text{ mg}} \times \frac{2 \text{ mg}}{\text{hr}} = 5 \text{ ml/hr}$$

DF × A × Or × U =
Ans

A × Or = Ans

E X A M P L E   7

Ordered: Furosemide 30 mg/hr IV
Available: Furosemide 100 mg in 250 ml of NS

1. Calculate the drip rate in gtt/min (15 gtt/ml).
2. Calculate the flow rate in ml/hr.

Pertinent information provided: 30 mg/hr; 100 mg/250 ml; 15 gtt/ml
Unit equivalency conversion: 60 min/hr
Desired units: (1) gtt/min (drip rate); (2) ml/h (flow rate)

DF = 15 gtt/ml
Or = 30 mg/hr
A = 100 mg/250 ml

CORRECT setup:

1. gtt/min:

$$\frac{15 \text{ gtt}}{\text{ml}} \times \frac{250 \text{ ml}}{100 \text{ mg}} \times \frac{30 \text{ mg}}{\text{hr}} \times \frac{\text{hr}}{60 \text{ min}} = 18.75 = 19 \text{ gtt/min}$$

DF × A × Or × U =
Ans

2. ml/hr:

$$\frac{250 \text{ ml}}{100 \text{ mg}} \times \frac{30 \text{ mg}}{\text{hr}} = 75 \text{ ml/hr}$$

A × Or = Ans

Total parenteral nutrition (TPN) is administered through a central line.

 Or × DF × U = Ans

 The cyclical administration of oncologic chemotherapeutic agents frequently requires a central line. Most chemotherapeutic agents are prepared by a pharmacist and delivered to the nursing unit or the provider for administration.

 Ord = 6 mg/kg/d

 A × Ord × U × BW = Ans

 Round the numbers to the nearest measurable unit.

 Continuous IV infusion orders are frequently based on the patient's body weight, for example, 0.05 mg/kg per min instead of 10 mg/min continuous IV.

 DF × A × Or × BW × Ot × U = Ans

E X A M P L E   1

Ordered: TPN induction with amino acid–dextrose solution 40 ml/hr for 24 hr

Available: Standard TPN Electrolytes (combined electrolyte solution) solution 1 L

Calculate the drip rate in gtt/min (15 gtt/ml).

Pertinent information provided: 40 ml/hr; 15 gtt/ml

Unit equivalency conversion: 60 min/hr

Desired unit: gtt/min

CORRECT setup:

$$\frac{40 \text{ ml}}{\text{hr}} \times \frac{15 \text{ gtt}}{\text{ml}} \times \frac{\text{hr}}{60 \text{ min}} = 10 \text{ gtt/min}$$

E X A M P L E   2

Ordered: 5-Fluorouracil 6 mg/kg per d (max 400 mg/d) IVSP for 3 d (first, second, and third d), pause 1 d (fourth day), and repeat the cycle on fifth and ninth days

Available: Fluorouracil 500 mg/10 ml in single-use vial

Calculate the number of ml/dose per d for a patient who weighs 98 lb.

Pertinent information provided: 6 mg/kg per d; 500 mg/10 ml; 400 mg/d; 98 lb

Unit equivalency conversion: 2.2 lb/kg

Desired unit: ml/d

CORRECT setup:

$$\frac{10 \text{ ml}}{500 \text{ mg}} \times \frac{6 \text{ mg}}{\text{kg} \cdot \text{d}} \times \frac{\text{kg}}{2.2 \text{ lb}} \times 98 \text{ lb} = 5.34 = 5.3 \text{ ml/d}$$

Round 5.34 to the nearest measurable unit of 5.3 ml; because a 10-ml (cc) syringe is not calibrated to allow the measurement of the volume to $\frac{1}{100}$ ml; rather, it is calibrated to measure to $\frac{1}{10}$ ml.

E X A M P L E   3

Ordered: Foscavir 60 mg/kg IV infusion over 8 hr/d for 3 wk, for a patient who weighs 90 kg

Available: Foscarnet sodium 24 mg/ml 500 ml bottle for IV infusion

1. Calculate the drip rate in gtt/min (20 gtt/ml).

2. Calculate flow rate in ml/hr.

Pertinent information provided: 60 mg/kg per dose; 90 kg; 24 mg/ml; 8 hr/dose; 20 gtt/ml

Unit equivalency conversion: 60 min/hr

Desired units: (1) gtt/min; (2) ml/hr

CORRECT setup:

1. gtt/min:

$$\frac{20 \text{ gtt}}{\text{ml}} \times \frac{\text{ml}}{24 \text{ mg}} \times \frac{60 \text{ mg}}{\text{kg} \cdot \text{dose}} \times 90 \text{ kg} \times \frac{\text{dose}}{8 \text{ hr}} \times \frac{\text{hr}}{60 \text{ min}} = 9.37 = 9 \text{ gtt/min}$$

2. ml/hr:

$$\frac{ml}{24 \text{ mg}} \times \frac{60 \text{ mg}}{\text{kg} \cdot \text{dose}} \times 90 \text{ kg} \times \frac{\text{dose}}{8 \text{ hr}} = 28.125 = 28 \text{ ml/hr}$$

You will need to round this answer to the nearest whole number, because the infusion pump will not allow you to enter decimal fractions.

EXAMPLE 4

Ordered: Cytovene 5 mg/kg IV over 60 min q12hr for 21 d
Available: Ganciclovir 500 mg/vial reconstituted with 10 ml of sterile water without parabens, and added to 100 ml of NS
Calculate the drip rate in gtt/min (15 gtt/ml).
Pertinent information provided: 60 min/dose; 100 ml/dose; 15 gtt/ml
Unit equivalency conversion: None needed
Desired unit: gtt/min

CORRECT setup:

$$\frac{15 \text{ gtt}}{\text{ml}} \times \frac{100 \text{ ml}}{\text{dose}} \times \frac{\text{dose}}{60 \text{ min}} = 25 \text{ gtt/min}$$

EXAMPLE 5

Ordered: Rocephin 1 gm over 30 min q12hr for 6 wk
Available: Rocephin (ceftriaxone sodium) 1 gm in 50 ml of D$_5$W
Calculate the drip rate in gtt/min (15 gtt/ml).
Pertinent information provided: 30 min/dose; 50 ml/dose; 15 gtt/ml
Unit equivalency conversion: None needed
Desired unit: gtt/min

CORRECT setup:

$$\frac{15 \text{ gtt}}{\text{ml}} \times \frac{50 \text{ ml}}{\text{dose}} \times \frac{\text{dose}}{30 \text{ min}} = 25 \text{ gtt/min}$$

A × Or × BW × Ot = Ans

Read the problem carefully. You do not need to calculate the dosage. The problem is asking you to calculate the drip rate to administer 100 ml of medication over 60 min.

DF = 15 gtt/ml
Ov = 100 ml/dose
Ot = 60 min/dose

DF × Ov × Ot = Ans

The placement of a central line in a patient who is scheduled to receive IV medication dosages at regular intervals over a significant period of time eliminates multiple peripheral catheter placements.

DF × Ov × Ot = Ans

Chapter Summary

If you are having difficulties in conceptualizing IV dosage calculation with DA, please review all the examples demonstrated in this chapter. Do not spend too much time with the examples provided under the central line section. There are additional examples of medication dosages requiring central lines in Chapter 12.

The following setup of the conversion factors can be used to calculate the drip rate (gtt/min) and the flow rate (ml/h):

Drop factor × Ordered volume
    × Ordered time = Drip rate

Ordered volume × Ordered time = Flow rate

✔ Do not introduce an error into the unit dimension in the process of transcribing the pertinent information provided in the problem; for example, under stress, μg, mg, gm, can look similar.

μgtt = micro drop

- ✔ Take care to set up conversion factors to allow unwanted units to cancel.
- ✔ Keep your desired dimension in the proper orientation of numerator and denominator; for example, ml/hr means that ml is the numerator, whereas hr will be the denominator in the setup.
- ✔ Remember to include the pertinent unit equivalency conversion factors in the setup.
- ✔ Be careful with questions that have multiple parts or subquestions that require you to carry an answer from one part to the next.
- ✔ Check your math.

PROBLEM SET	PROBLEM SET ANSWERS
1. Ordered: NS 1 L at 40 ml/hr Calculate the drip rate in μgtt/min. *60 gtt/mL*	1. 40 μgtt/min
2. Ordered: NS with D_5W 500 ml over 2 hr Calculate the drip rate in gtt/min (15 gtt/ml).	2. 62.5 = 63 gtt/min
3. Ordered: Heparin 1000 U/hr continuous IV Available: Heparin 20,000 U in 500 ml of D_5W (dextrose in water) Calculate the drip rate in μgtt/min.	3. 25 μgtt/min
4. Ordered: ½ NS 1 L over 1 hr Calculate the drip rate in gtt/min (10 gtt/ml).	4. 166.6 = 167 gtt/min
5. Ordered: Acyclovir 100 mg/500 ml over 1 hr Calculate the drip rate in gtt/min (15 gtt/ml).	5. 125 gtt/min

PROBLEM SET	PROBLEM SET ANSWERS

6. Ordered: Adenosine 6 mg IVSP now
    Available: Adenosine 3 mg/ml vial
    Calculate the number of ml/dose.

6. 2 ml/dose

7. Ordered: Albuminar 25% 100 ml over 1 hr
    Calculate the drip rate in μgtt/min.

7. 100 μgtt/min

8. Ordered: Adenosine 12 mg IVSP now
    Available: Adenocard 2 mg/ml vial.
    Calculate the number of ml/dose.

8. 6 ml/dose

9. Ordered: Calan 5 mg IVSP q6hr
    Available: Verapamil HCl 5 mg/2 ml
    Calculate the number of ml/dose.

9. 2 ml/dose

10. Ordered: Sulfamethoxazole and trimethoprim 160/800 mg in 50 ml of
    NS IVPB over 30 min q12hr
    Available: Sulfamethoxazole/trimethoprin 80/400 in 5-ml vial.
    Calculate the drip rate in gtt/min (15 gtt/ml).

10. 25 gtt/min

11. Ordered: Procan IV at 20 mg/min
    Available: Procainamide HCl 2 gm in 500 ml of D_5W
    Calculate the flow rate (ml/hr).

11. 300 ml/hr

PROBLEM SET	PROBLEM SET ANSWERS
12. Ordered: Norcuron 0.06 mg/kg/hr continuous IV for a patient who weighs 148 lb Available: Vecuronium bromide 50 mg in 100 ml D_5W Calculate the drip rate in μgtt/min.	12. 8 μgtt/min
13. Ordered: Meperidine 50 mg IVSP q.i.d. p.r.n. Available: Meperidine 100 mg/ml Calculate the number of ml/dose.	13. ½ ml/dose
14. Ordered: Diphenhydramine 50 mg IVSP Available: Diphenhydramine 10 mg/ml Calculate the number of ml/dose.	14. 5 ml/dose
15. Ordered: Ca-glu 2 gm IVPB at 1 gm/hr Available: Calcium gluconate 1 gm/100 ml NS a. Calculate the drip rate in μgtt/min. b. Calculate the total time necessary for infusion.	15. a. 100 μgtt/min b. 2-hr total infusion time
16. Ordered: Lidocaine 4 mg/min Available: Lidocaine 2 gm in 500 ml of D_5W Calculate the drip rate in gtt/min (15 gtt/ml).	16. 15 gtt/min

PROBLEM SET	PROBLEM SET ANSWERS

17. Ordered: Flagyl 500 mg in 50 ml of NS IVPB over 30 min q.i.d.
Calculate the drip rate in μgtt/min.

17. 100 μgtt/min

18. Ordered: Premarin 25 mg IVSP b.i.d.
Available: Premarin (conjugated estrogen) 25 mg/ml vial
Calculate the number of ml/dose.

18. 1 ml/dose

19. Ordered: Morphine sulfate 8 mg IVSP q4hr p.r.n.
Available: Morphine sulfate 3 mg/ml Tubex
Calculate the number of ml/dose.

19. 2.67 = 2.7 ml/dose

20. Ordered: Morphine sulfate 0.05 mg/kg/hr continuous IV for a patient
who weighs 228 lb
Available: Morphine sulfate 100 mg/250 ml of D₅W
Calculate the drip rate μgtt/min.

20. 12.95 = 13 μgtt/min

21. Ordered: Pitressin 20 U IVPB over 20 min for induction, then 0.2 U/min
continuous IV infusion for maintenance
Available: Vasopressin 100 U in 250 ml D₅W
Calculate the flow rates (ml/hr) for induction and maintenance.

21. Induction = 150 ml/hr
Maintenance = 30 ml/hr

PROBLEM SET	PROBLEM SET ANSWERS

22. Ordered: Zantac 50 mg IVSP bolus
     Available: Ranitidine 25 mg/ml in 40-ml vial
     Calculate the number of ml/dose.

22. 2 ml/dose

23. Ordered: Zantac 6.25 mg/hr continuous IV infusion for 24 hr
     Available: Ranitidine 150 mg in 500 ml of D$_5$W
     Calculate the flow rate (ml/hr).

23. $20.8 = 21$ ml/hr

24. Ordered: Zantac 10 mg/hr continuous IV infusion for 24 hr
     Available: Ranitidine 300 mg in 500 ml D$_5$W
     a.   Calculate the drip rate in gtt/min (10 gtt/ml).
     b.   Would you rather use a microdrop administrator for this order?

24. a. $2.8 = 3$ gtt/min
     b. Yes. 17 μgtt/min
     will be easier to count
     in microdrops.

25. Ordered: Pepcid 20 mg IVSP q12hr
     Available: Famotidine 10 mg/ml 2-ml vial
     Calculate the number of ml/dose.

25. 2 ml/dose

26. Ordered: Cefizox 2 gm IVPB over 10 min q8hr
     Available: Ceftizoxime sodium 2 gm reconstituted with 13 ml of sterile
     water added into 100 ml of NS
     Calculate the drip rate in gtt/min (10 gtt/ml).

26. 100 gtt/min

PROBLEM SET	PROBLEM SET ANSWERS

27. Ordered: Claforan 2 gm IVPB q.i.d.
     Available: Cefotaxime sodium 1-gm vial
     Calculate the number of vial/dose.

27. 2 vial/dose

28. Ordered: Mefoxin 1 gm continuous IV infusion q.i.d.
     Available: Cefoxitin sodium 2 gm/100 ml D_5NS infusion bottle
     a. Calculate the flow rate for this order (ml/hr).
     b. Calculate the number of bottle/d.

28. a. 8.3 ml = 8 ml/hr
     b. 2 bottle/d

29. Ordered: Cefotan 2 gm IVPB over 30 min b.i.d.
     Available: Cefotetan disodium 10 gm/100-ml vial
     Calculate the number of ml/24 hr.

29. 40 ml/24 hr

30. Ordered: Cefotan 2 gm IVPB over 15 min b.i.d.
     Available: Cefotetan disodium 4 gm/100 ml of D_5W
     a. Calculate the flow rate.
     b. Calculate the drip rate in gtt/min (15 gtt/ml).

30. a. 200 ml/hr
     b. 50 gtt/min

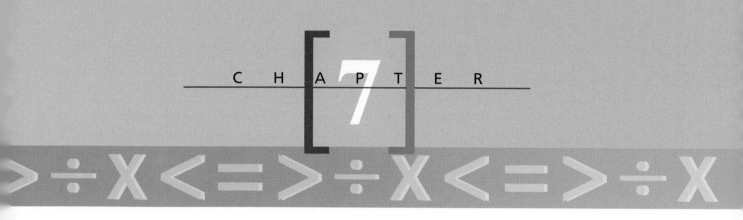

Pediatric Population: Medication Calculation Using Dimensional Analysis

INTRODUCTION

In this chapter, the process of implementing dimensional analysis (DA) to calculate medication dosages for the pediatric population will be demonstrated. The focus of the chapter is on dosage calculations, but a brief discussion of medication administration issues within the pediatric population will be provided.

The examples of dosage calculation problems will be presented as scenarios, breaking away from the previous ordered/available format. You will need to read each problem carefully, analyze it, and decide what the problem is asking you to solve. You will continue to find information in the form of Keys, Hints, Pearls, and Warnings in the outside column, along with highlights on how to solve each problem.

LEARNING OBJECTIVES

By the end of this chapter, you will be able to:

- Explain pediatric dosage calculations based on body weight (BW)

- Review pediatric dosage calculations based on body surface area (BSA)

- Use DA in calculating minimum fluid requirements

- Implement DA in calculating caloric requirements

- Employ DA in calculating pediatric parenteral medication dosages

Body weight can be mea-
sured in lb or kg.

CALCULATIONS FOR ADMINISTRATION OF PEDIATRIC MEDICATIONS

A few examples of medication dosages based on patient body weight (BW) have appeared in Chapters 5 and 6. Pediatric medication dosages, however, are based mainly on patient BW. A few medications are given based on BSA, and they will also be discussed.

Implementing DA in pediatric medication dosages requires inclusion of the patient's BW as a conversion factor. Most pediatric dosages are ordered in a specified amount, for example, Suprax (cefixime) suspension ½ tsp q.d. for 10 d; or, they are based on a reference dose schedule, such as mg/kg per dose, μg/kg per d, U/kg per min, ml/kg per hr, where kg is used for the patient's BW. Therefore, in solving pediatric dosage problems, be wary of how the dose is ordered, because you will need to use the same unit in your final DA setup.

Dosage Calculation Based on Body Weight

The following pediatric dosage orders are based on the patient's BW.

Most reference doses are based on BW in kg. Septra is one of the few exceptions.

(Ord) = 5 ml/22 lb

Ord × BW = Ans

E X A M P L E   1

Septra (trimethoprim; sulfamethoxazole) suspension was ordered for Mark, who weighs 44 lb. The reference dose (Ordered Reference Dose) for Septra suspension is 5 ml/22 lb PO b.i.d. Calculate the number of ml/dose.

Pertinent information provided: 44 lb; 5 ml/22 lb (Ord)
Unit equivalency conversion: None needed
Desired unit: ml/dose

CORRECT setup:

$$\frac{5 \text{ ml}}{22 \text{ lb}} \times 44 \text{ lb} = 10 \text{ ml}$$

E X A M P L E   2

The reference dose for Ceclor* (cefaclor) is 40 mg/kg per d PO t.i.d. (maximum 500 mg/dose). Jane weighs 36 lb. Available is Ceclor 250 mg/5 ml.

1. Calculate the number of mg/dose.
2. Calculate the number of ml/dose.

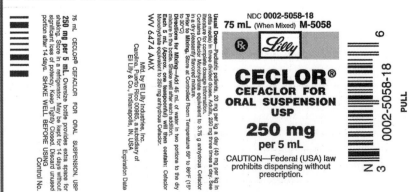

---

* Ceclor® is a registered trademark of Eli Lilly and Company.

Pertinent information provided: 40 mg/kg per d; 3 dose/d; 36 lb; 250 mg/5 ml
Unit equivalency conversion: 2.2 lb/kg
Desired units: (1) mg/dose; (2) ml/dose

CORRECT setup:

1. mg/dose:

$$\frac{40\ mg}{kg \cdot d} \times \frac{d}{3\ dose} \times \frac{kg}{2.2\ lb} \times 36\ lb = 218\ mg/dose$$

2. ml/dose:

$$\frac{5\ ml}{250\ mg} \times \frac{40\ mg}{kg \cdot d} \times \frac{d}{3\ dose} \times \frac{kg}{2.2\ lb} \times 36\ lb = 4.36 = 4\ ml/dose$$

In reality, the answer will be rounded to 4 ml/dose for a practical reason (easy measurement) as long as the dosage falls within the therapeutic range, that is, the addition of 0.3 ml will not make any difference in the efficacy of the medication.

 Os = Ordered dose schedule
Ord = 40 mg/kg per d
Os = t.i.d. = 3 dose/d
A = 250 mg/5 ml

 Round the numbers to the nearest measurable unit, e.g., ml, tsp.

 Ord × Os × U × BW = Ans

 A × Ord × Os × U × BW = Ans

 If you have any doubt about the therapeutic range (and toxicity level) of a medication, double-check with a pharmacist.

EXAMPLE 3

Jim is to receive Lorabid 30 mg/kg per d PO b.i.d. Jim is 3 years old and weighs 40 lb. Loracarbef suspension is available in 100 mg/5 ml. Calculate the number of ml/dose.
Pertinent information provided: 30 mg/kg per d; 2 dose/d; 40 lb; 100 mg/5 ml
Unit equivalency conversion: 2.2 lb/kg
Desired unit: ml/dose

 Ord = 30 mg/kg per d
Os = 2 dose/d
A = 100 mg/5 ml

CORRECT setup:

$$\frac{5\ ml}{100\ mg} \times \frac{30\ mg}{kg \cdot d} \times \frac{d}{2\ dose} \times \frac{kg}{2.2\ lb} \times 40\ lb = 13.63$$
$$= 13.6 = 13.5\ ml/dose$$

 A × Ord × Os × U × BW = Ans

EXAMPLE 4

Suprax suspension was ordered for the infant Alyssa, who weighs 14 lb. The reference dose for Suprax is 8 mg/kg per d PO q.d. (max 400 mg/dose). You have cefixime 100 mg/5-ml suspension. Calculate the number of ml/dose for Alyssa.
Pertinent information provided: 8 mg/kg per d; 1 dose/d; 14 lb; 100 mg/5 ml
Unit equivalency conversion: 2.2 lb/kg
Desired unit: ml/dose

 Ord = 8 mg/kg per d
Os = 1 dose/d
A = 100 mg/5 ml

CORRECT setup:

$$\frac{5\ ml}{100\ mg} \times \frac{8\ mg}{kg \cdot d} \times \frac{d}{1\ dose} \times \frac{kg}{2.2\ lb} \times 14\ lb = 2.54 = 2.5\ ml/dose$$

 A × Ord × Os × U × BW = Ans

You will round the answer to 2.5, because in dosage administration it is impossible to measure 2.54 ml using a standard 5-ml (cc) syringe.

Ord = 50 mg/kg per d
Os = 4 dose/d
A = 125 mg/5 ml

E X A M P L E   5

The Penicillin V potassium reference dose is 50 mg/kg per d PO q.i.d. Sam weighs 28 lb. Available is V-Cillin K* 125 mg/5 ml. Calculate the number of ml/dose.

Pertinent information provided: 50 mg/kg per d; 4 dose/d; 28 lb; 125 mg/5 ml
Unit equivalency conversion: 2.2 lb/kg
Desired unit: mg/dose

CORRECT setup:

A × Ord × Os × U × BW = Ans

$$\frac{5 \text{ ml}}{125 \text{ mg}} \times \frac{50 \text{ mg}}{\text{kg} \cdot \text{d}} \times \frac{\text{d}}{4 \text{ dose}} \times \frac{\text{kg}}{2.2 \text{ lb}} \times 28 \text{ lb} = 6.36 = 6 \text{ ml/dose}$$

E X A M P L E   6

Magnesium hydroxide 2 tsp PO q.h.s. was ordered for Garvey, who weighs 46 lb. The reference dose for milk of magnesia is 40 mg/kg per dose. Milk of magnesia is available in 80 mg/ml. Is the order appropriate for Garvey?
Pertinent information provided: 40 mg/kg per dose; 46 lb; 2 tsp/dose; 80 mg/ml
Unit equivalency conversion: 2.2 lb/kg; 5 ml/tsp
Desired units: (1) mg/dose as ordered for Garvey; (2) mg/dose indicated in reference dose

Ord = 40 mg/kg per dose
O = 2 tsp/dose
A = 80 mg/ml

CORRECT setup:

1. mg/dose ordered:

A × U × O = Ans

$$\frac{80 \text{ mg}}{\text{ml}} \times \frac{5 \text{ ml}}{\text{tsp}} \times \frac{2 \text{ tsp}}{\text{dose}} = 800 \text{ mg/dose}$$

2. mg/dose according to the reference dose:

Ord × U × BW = Ans

$$\frac{40 \text{ mg}}{\text{kg} \cdot \text{dose}} \times \frac{\text{kg}}{2.2 \text{ lb}} \times 46 \text{ lb} = 836 \text{ mg/dose}$$

The 800 mg/dose ordered is close to the reference dose of 836 mg/dose.

Answer: The order is appropriate for Garvey.

---

* V-Cillin K® is a registered trademark of Eli Lilly and Company.

EXAMPLE   7

The reference limit for Omnipen is 50 to 100 mg/kg per d PO given q.i.d. (max 2 gm/d). The order for your teenage patient, Zachary, who weighs 122 lb, is to give 500 mg PO q.i.d. Available is ampicillin 250 mg/5 ml. Does this order fall within the reference limit?

Pertinent information provided: 50 to 100 mg/kg per d; 4 dose/d; 122 lb
Unit equivalency conversion: 2.2 lb/kg
Desired unit: mg/dose at lower and upper limits

CORRECT setup:

1. Lower reference limit:

$$\frac{50 \text{ mg}}{\text{kg} \cdot \text{d}} \times \frac{\text{d}}{4 \text{ dose}} \times \frac{\text{kg}}{2.2 \text{ lb}} \times 122 \text{ lb} = 693 \text{ mg/dose}$$

2. Upper reference limit:

$$\frac{100 \text{ mg}}{\text{kg} \cdot \text{d}} \times \frac{\text{d}}{4 \text{ dose}} \times \frac{\text{kg}}{2.2 \text{ lb}} \times 122 \text{ lb} = 1386 \text{ mg/dose}$$

Answer: No, the 500 mg/dose falls below the lower limit, that is, 500 mg < 693 mg < 1386 mg/dose. However, 500 mg/dose × 4 doses/d = 2000 mg/d and is the maximum dosage for ampicillin. Therefore, the ordered dosage is correct.

 The reference dose and limits serve as guidelines to prevent over- and underdosage, that is, achieve efficacy without toxicity.

 1. and 2. Ord × Os × U × BW = Ans

 Complete the problem set for the upper and lower reference limits. The ordered dose should fall within this range.

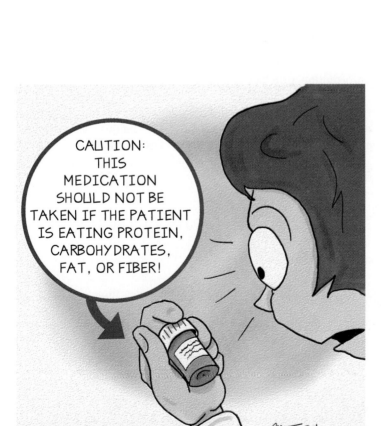

Ord range = 0.25 to
1.0 mg/kg per d
Os = 4 dose/d
O = ½ supp/dose
A = 12.5 mg/supp

EXAMPLE   8

Joey is a 15-month-old baby who weighs 25 lb. He is vomiting and cannot keep food down. The provider has ordered Phenergan 12.5 mg suppositories (supp), ½ supp PR q.i.d. p.r.n. The reference dose for Phenergan is 0.25 to 1 mg/kg per dose q.i.d. p.r.n. (max 50 mg/dose). Available are promethazine 12.5-mg supp. Is the ordered dose within the reference limit?

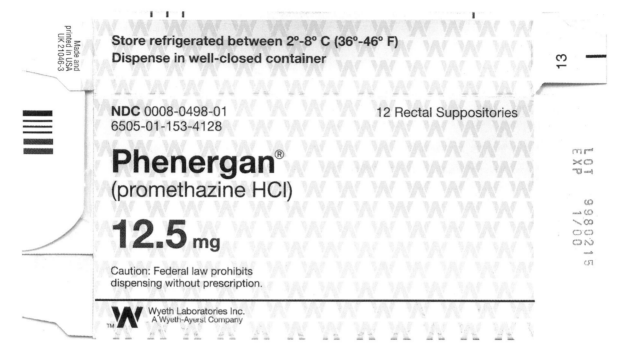

Store refrigerated between 2°-8° C (36°-46° F)
Dispense in well-closed container

NDC 0008-0498-01
6505-01-153-4128

12 Rectal Suppositories

Phenergan®
(promethazine HCl)

12.5 mg

Caution: Federal law prohibits
dispensing without prescription.

W Wyeth Laboratories Inc.
™ A Wyeth-Ayerst Company

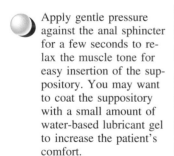

Apply gentle pressure against the anal sphincter for a few seconds to relax the muscle tone for easy insertion of the suppository. You may want to coat the suppository with a small amount of water-based lubricant gel to increase the patient's comfort.

A × O = Ans

Ord × U × BW = Ans

Pertinent information provided: 0.25 to 1.0 mg/kg per d; 4 dose/d; 25 lb; ½ supp/dose; 12.5 mg/supp

Unit equivalency conversion: 2.2 lb/kg

Desired units: (1) mg/dose ordered for Joey; (2) mg/dose at the lower reference limit; (3) mg/dose at the upper reference limit

CORRECT setup:

1. mg/dose ordered for Joey:

$$\frac{12.5 \text{ mg}}{\text{supp}} \times \frac{1 \text{ supp}}{2 \text{ dose}} = 6.25 \text{ mg/dose ordered for little Joey}$$

2. mg/dose at the lower reference limit:

$$\frac{0.25 \text{ mg}}{\text{kg} \cdot \text{dose}} \times \frac{\text{kg}}{2.2 \text{ lb}} \times 25 \text{ lb} = 2.8 \text{ mg/dose at the lower limit}$$

3. mg/dose at the upper reference limit:

$$\frac{1.0 \text{ mg}}{\text{kg} \cdot \text{dose}} \times \frac{\text{kg}}{2.2 \text{ lb}} \times 25 \text{ lb} = 11.4 \text{ mg/dose at the upper limit}$$

The ordered dose falls within the reference limit, that is, 2.8 mg < 6.25 mg < 11.4 mg/dose.

Dosage Calculation Based on Body Surface Area

To calculate medication dosages using BSA, you will need to convert your patient's ht and BW into BSA. To do this, you will use a nomogram. The following is a West nomogram for BSA. Depending on where you work, you may have a different version of the nomogram (Fig. 7–1) for BSA (see Appendix for Du Bois' nomogram).

 The unit of measure for body surface area is m² (squared meter, that is, m × m). A meter (m) is a linear measurement in a metric unit.

 Medication orders using BSA are given in reference doses of mg/m². Extremely toxic medications, such as antineoplastic agents, are calculated based on BSA.

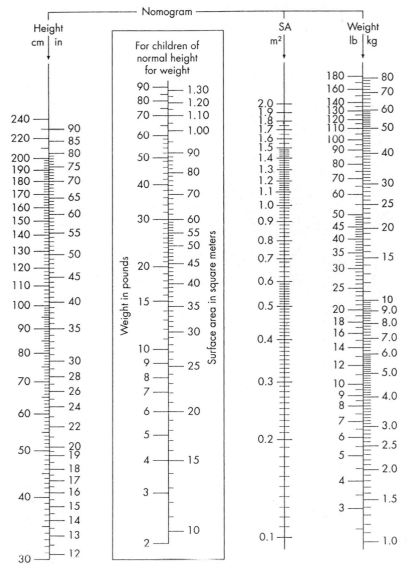

Figure 7–1 *A West body surface area nomogram. (From Olsen JL, Ablon LJ, Giangrasso AP. Medical Dosage Calculations, 6th ed. Reading, MA, Addison-Wesley, 1995, p. A-29. Redrawn from Behrman RE, Kliegman RM, Arvin AM, eds.* Nelson Textbook of Pediatrics, 15th ed. *Philadelphia, WB Saunders, 1996, p. 2079, with permission.)*

The West nomogram comes with a calibrated BSA scale for children of normal ht for wt. It is easier on your eyes if you use a transparent ruler to determine BSA from a nomogram.

The reference dose based on BSA is presented as mg/m^2. The following are examples using DA for dosage calculations of orders based on BSA.

To convert ht and wt to BSA:

- Find the patient's ht on the ht scale.
- Find the patient's wt on the wt scale.
- Plot a straight line using the two points.
- The intersection on the BSA line is the corresponding BSA value for the patient.

E X A M P L E   1

Sydney, a 4-year-old patient, is 3 ft tall and weighs 53 lb. She is receiving an antineoplastic-antibiotic derivative on a weekly basis. The order is for Adriamycin (doxorubicin HCl) 20 mg/m^2 per dose. The order is given to the pharmacy, and the medication is delivered premixed. Calculate Sydney's Adriamycin dosage in mg/dose.

From the nomogram:
3 ft, 53 lb = 0.82 m^2

Pertinent information provided: 3 ft; 53 lb; 20 mg/m^2 per dose
Unit equivalency conversion: From the nomogram
Desired unit: mg/dose

Ord = 20 mg/m^2 per dose

CORRECT setup:

$$\frac{20 \text{ mg}}{\text{m}^2 \cdot \text{dose}} \times 0.82 \text{ m}^2 = 16.4 \text{ mg/dose}$$

Ord × BSA = Ans

E X A M P L E   2 a

Cortisone was ordered for Waverley (30 mo), who weighs 24 lb and measures 28 inches. The reference order for cortisone acetate is 20 mg/m^2 per d PO q.i.d. Cortisone acetate is available in 5-mg tab. The provider has ordered Cortone Acetate 5-mg tab, ½ tab (crushed) q.i.d. Is this order appropriate for Waverley?

From the nomogram:
28 in, 24 lb = 0.475 m^2

Ord = 20 mg/m^2 per d
Os = 4 dose/d
A = 5 mg/tab

Pertinent information provided: 28 inches and 24 lb; 20 mg/m^2 per d; 4 dose/d; 5 mg/tab
Unit equivalency conversion: From the nomogram
Desired unit: tab/dose

Give crushed medications mixed in a small amount of applesauce, but be aware that food adversion may result.

CORRECT setup:

$$\frac{\text{tab}}{5 \text{ mg}} \times \frac{20 \text{ mg}}{\text{m}^2 \cdot \text{d}} \times \frac{\text{d}}{4 \text{ dose}} \times 0.475 \text{ m}^2 = 0.475 = \text{½ tab/dose}$$

A × Ord × Os × BSA = Ans

The provider has rounded to the nearest measurable unit of tab, that is, ½ tab for this order. It is appropriate for Waverley.

E X A M P L E   2 b

Waverley was vomiting and could not keep the ordered cortisone down, so the order was changed to IM administration. The reference dose for IM cortisone acetate is 12.5 mg/m^2 per d IM qAM. Cortisone acetate is available in a 50 mg/ml strength. Calculate the number of ml/dose.

BSA from example 2a = 0.475 m^2
Ord = 12.5 mg/m^2/d
Os = 1 dose/d
A = 50 mg/ml

Pertinent information provided: 28 inches and 24 lb (30 mo) (see example 2a); 12.5 mg/m^2 per d; 1 dose/d; 50 mg/ml
Unit equivalency conversion: From the nomogram
Desired unit: ml/dose

CORRECT setup:

$$\frac{1 \text{ ml}}{50 \text{ mg}} \times \frac{12.5 \text{ mg}}{\text{m}^2 \cdot \text{d}} \times \frac{\text{d}}{1 \text{ dose}} \times 0.475 \text{ m}^2 = 0.12 \text{ ml/dose}$$

Tuberculin syringes are calibrated to measure to 0.01 of a ml. Therefore, you can use a tuberculin syringe to measure this dose.

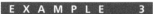

EXAMPLE 3

The reference dose for Videx is as follows:

BSA < 0.4 m², give 25 mg PO b.i.d.

BSA 0.5 to 0.7 m², give 50 mg PO b.i.d.

BSA 0.8 to 1.0 m², give 75 mg PO b.i.d.

BSA 1.1 to 1.4 m², give 100 mg PO b.i.d.

John, who is 6 years old, weighs 40 lb and measures 45 inches in ht. Available is Videx (didanosine) powder to be reconstituted to 100 mg/5 ml. Calculate the number of ml/dose.

    Pertinent information provided: Reference dose schedule; 100 mg/5 ml; 40 lb, 45 inches

    Unit equivalency conversion: From the nomogram

    Desired unit: ml/dose

CORRECT setup:

From the nomogram, John's BSA = 0.75 m². According to the reference dose schedule, John will need 50 mg PO b.i.d.

$$\frac{5 \text{ ml}}{100 \text{ mg}} \times \frac{50 \text{ mg}}{\text{dose}} = 2.5 \text{ ml/dose}$$

EXAMPLE 4

The order for the treatment of lead poisoning is calcium EDTA (ethylenediaminetetraacetic acid) 1000 mg/m² per d in a continuous IV infusion for 3 days. Tommy weighs 38 lb and measures 42 inches. Edetate calcium disodium is available in a 200 mg/ml 5-ml vial. Calculate the number of ml of calcium EDTA for the 3-d dose.

    Pertinent information provided: 1000 mg/m² per d; 38 lb, 42 inches; 200 mg/ml; 3 d

    Unit equivalency conversion: From the nomogram

    Desired unit: ml

CORRECT setup:

$$\frac{\text{ml}}{200 \text{ mg}} \times \frac{1000 \text{ mg}}{\text{m}^2 \cdot \text{d}} \times 3 \text{ d} \times 0.72 \text{ m}^2 = 10.8 \text{ ml}$$

EXAMPLE 5

Roferon-A 2 million U/m² per d SQ was ordered for Alice who weighs 68 lb and is of normal ht. This Interferon alpha-2a recombinant is available in a vial containing 3 million U/ml. Calculate the number of ml/d.

A × Ord × Os × BSA = Ans

Ord = as listed

BSA from the nomogram: 40 lb, 45 in = 0.75 m²

A = 50 mg/tab

Shake a suspension prior to administration.

From the reference dose schedule, with a BSA of 0.75 m², the patient will require 50 mg PO b.i.d.

A × O = Ans

Ord = 1000 mg/m² per d
Ot = 3 d
A = 200 mg/ml

BSA from the nomogram for 38 lb, 42 in. = 0.72 m²

A × Ord × Ot × BSA = Ans

Ord = 2 mU/m² per d
A = 6 mU/ml

The BSA from the nomogram for children = 1.075 m².

Reference dose for fluids:
- 100 ml/kg per d for the first 10 kg
- 50 ml/kg per d for the second 10 kg
- 20 ml/kg per d for each additional kg

Ord × BW = Ans
The first 10 kg will use 100 ml/kg per d, the second 10 kg will use 50 ml/kg per d, and the remaining 3.6 kg will use 20 ml/kg per d.

CORRECT setup:

Convert BW to kg:

$$52 \text{ lb} \times \frac{\text{kg}}{2.2 \text{ lb}} = 23.6 \text{ kg}$$

$$\frac{100 \text{ ml}}{\text{kg} \cdot \text{d}} \times 10 \text{ kg} = 1000 \text{ ml/d}$$

$$\frac{50 \text{ ml}}{\text{kg} \cdot \text{d}} \times 10 \text{ kg} = 500 \text{ ml/d}$$

$$\frac{20 \text{ ml}}{\text{kg} \cdot \text{d}} \times 3.6 \text{ kg} = 72 \text{ ml/d}$$

Total fluid requirement for 24 hr = 1000 + 500 + 72 ml = 1572 ml/d

E X A M P L E 4

Chris was ordered Pedialyte ad lib, for 2 d for replacement of fluids and electrolytes lost as a result of diarrhea and vomiting. She weighs 36 lb and is 3 years old. Calculate the minimum amount of fluid needed in ml/d for Chris.

Pertinent information provided: 36 lb; reference fluid dose
Unit equivalency conversion: 2.2 lb/kg (22 lb/10 kg)
Desired unit: ml/d

Ad lib. orders do not have a dosing schedule; they stipulate giving as much as the patient desires to consume.

Use 22 lb = 10 kg

From Example 3, 22 lb will require 1000 ml. The remaining 14 lb will require 318 ml/d.

BW × U × Ord = Ans

CORRECT setup:

The first 22 lb requires 1000 ml (see Example 3).

$$36 \text{ lb} - 22 \text{ lb} = 14 \text{ lb} \times \frac{\text{kg}}{2.2 \text{ lb}} \times \frac{50 \text{ ml}}{\text{kg d}} = 318 \text{ ml/d}$$

Ans = 1000 ml + 318 ml = 1318 ml/d

CALCULATIONS FOR ADMINISTRATION OF PEDIATRIC PARENTERAL MEDICATIONS

The smaller body size of pediatric patients requires extra safety measures in the administration of fluids. Additionally, their body systems are not able to function in the same way as their adult counterparts. Fluids and parenteral medications given at a rapid rate or in large quantities can cause toxicity that is potentially life threatening.

Intravenous administration of fluids and medications to pediatric patients is accomplished via a small-volume delivery system (Fig. 7–2), such as Buretrol, Volutrol, or Soluset. This type of system serves as an extension of the primary system, in as much as the fluid from the primary system is channeled into the small-volume delivery system (SVDS). Calibration marks on the

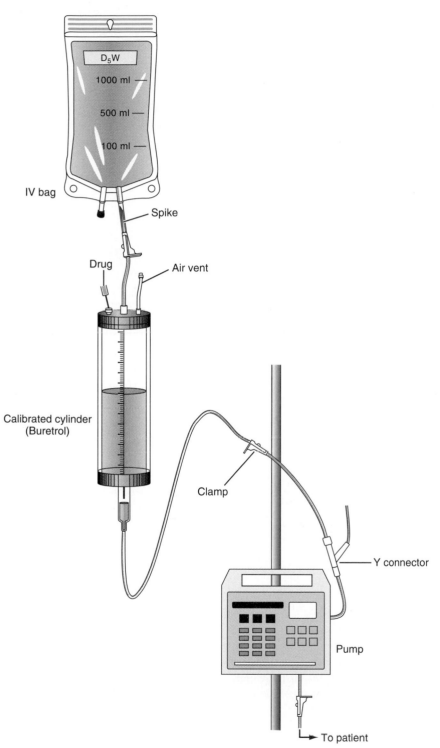

Figure 7–2 *Intravenous administration using small-volume delivery system—Buretrol. (Modified from Kee JL, Marshall SM.* Clinical Calculations, *2nd ed. Philadelphia, WB Saunders, 1992, pp. 125, 131, 134, with permission.)*

SVDS = Small-volume delivery system. The SVDS prevents fluid volume overload.

To avoid potential toxicity with pediatric dosages, do not round numbers higher. Round numbers lower, to the nearest measurable unit.

A × O = Ans

Ord = 2 mg/kg per dose
A = 50 mg/ml

You can choose to start the setup with the patient's BW.

BW × U × Ord × A = Ans

or

A × Ord × U × BW = Ans

Ord = 150 U/kg per dose
A = 2000 U/ml

A × Ord × U × BW = Ans

SVDS allow the nurse to measure volume in ml and cc prior to administration. In addition to fluids, small volumes of medications are injected directly into the SVDS for administration.

The following examples employ DA to calculate dosages for parenteral administration of pediatric medications to this population.

E X A M P L E   1

Aquamephyton 0.5 mg SQ or IM is the standing order for neonates within 1 hr after birth. Available is phytonadione 2 mg/ml. Calculate the number of ml/dose.

Pertinent information provided: 0.5 mg/dose; 2 mg/ml
Unit equivalency conversion: None needed
Desired unit: ml/dose

CORRECT setup:

$$\frac{ml}{2\ \cancel{mg}} \times \frac{0.5\ \cancel{mg}}{dose} = 0.25\ ml/dose$$

E X A M P L E   2

For preoperative sedation, Nembutal 2 mg/kg per dose IM is ordered for Jacky, who weighs 32 lb. Pentobarbital sodium is available in a 50-mg/ml vial. Calculate the number of ml/dose for Jacky.

Pertinent information provided: 2 mg/kg per dose; 32 lb; 50 mg/ml
Unit equivalency conversion: 2.2 lb/kg
Desired unit: ml/dose

CORRECT setup:

$$32\ \cancel{lb} \times \frac{kg}{2.2\ \cancel{lb}} \times \frac{2\ \cancel{mg}}{kg \cdot dose} \times \frac{ml}{50\ \cancel{mg}} = 0.5818 = 0.58\ ml/dose$$

or

$$\frac{ml}{50\ \cancel{mg}} \times \frac{2\ \cancel{mg}}{kg \cdot dose} \times \frac{kg}{2.2\ \cancel{lb}} \times 32\ \cancel{lb} = 0.5818 = 0.58\ ml/dose$$

E X A M P L E   3

Epogen 150 U/kg per dose SQ is ordered for Ludwig, who weighs 54 lb. Available is epoetin alfa 2000 U/ml. Calculate the number of ml/dose.

Pertinent information provided: 150 U/kg per dose; 54 lb; 2000 U/ml
Unit equivalency conversion: 2.2 lb/kg
Desired unit: ml/dose

CORRECT setup:

$$\frac{ml}{2000\ \cancel{U}} \times \frac{150\ \cancel{U}}{kg \cdot dose} \times \frac{kg}{2.2\ \cancel{lb}} \times 54\ \cancel{lb} = 1.84 = 1.8\ ml/dose$$

In addition to the SVDS, use a small-volume IV fluid unit bag to avoid fluid volume overload.

EXAMPLE 4

The reference dose for Dolophine is 0.7 mg/kg per d SC given q.i.d. Newborn Emma weighs 5 lb 8 oz. Available is Dolophine (methadone HCl) 10 mg/ml. Calculate the number of ml/dose.

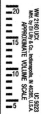 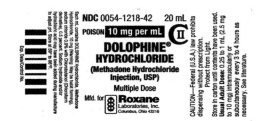

Pertinent information provided: 0.7 mg/kg per d; 4 dose per d; 5 lb 8 oz; 10 mg/ml
Unit equivalency conversion: 2.2 lb/kg; 16 oz/lb
Desired unit: ml/dose

CORRECT setup:

BW: $8 \text{ oz} \times \dfrac{\text{lb}}{16 \text{ oz}} = 0.5 \text{ lb} + 5 \text{ lb} = 5.5 \text{ lb}$

$\dfrac{0.7 \text{ mg}}{\text{kg} \cdot \text{d}} \times \dfrac{\text{d}}{4 \text{ dose}} \times \dfrac{\text{ml}}{10 \text{ mg}} \times \dfrac{\text{kg}}{2.2 \text{ lb}} \times 5.5 \text{ lb} = 0.043 = 0.04 \text{ ml/dose}$

Ord = 0.7 mg/kg per d
Os = 4 dose/d
A = 10 mg/ml

Convert BW to lb.

Ord × Os × A × U × BW = Ans

EXAMPLE 5

Johnny, a 9-year-old boy, is to receive Amikin 18 mg/kg per d in 50 ml of NS IV over 30 min in t.i.d. doses. Johnny weighs 79 lb. You have amikacin sulfate 250 mg/ml in a 2-ml vial.

1. Calculate the drip rate in µgtt/min and the flow rate in ml/hr.
2. Would you use an SVDS for this order?

Read the problem carefully. This is a straightforward drip-rate and flow-rate problem.

DF = 60 µgtt/ml
Oft = 50 ml/30 min

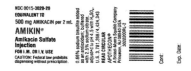

Pertinent information provided: 50 ml/30 min
Unit equivalency conversion: 60 min/hr; 60 µgtt/ml
Desired units: (1) µgtt/min; (2) ml/hr

CORRECT setup:

1. µgtt/min:

$\dfrac{60 \text{ µgtt}}{\text{ml}} \times \dfrac{50 \text{ ml}}{30 \text{ min}} = 100 \text{ µgtt/min}$

DF × Oft = Ans

Chapter Summary

This chapter has presented the fundamentals of pediatric medication dosage administration. In administering medication to the pediatric population, special care is needed to accommodate smaller body size and physiologic states that differ from those of adults. To avoid potential toxicity from overdosage and inefficacy from underdosage, most pediatric medications are calculated based on either the BW or the BSA. Although BSA is more accurate than BW, most available reference dosages of medications in the *Physicians' Desk Reference* (PDR) are based on the patient's BW. Dosage questions based on BSA will provide you either with the patient's BSA or with sufficient information for you to extract the BSA from the nomogram.

Additionally, the youngest members of the pediatric population, that is, neonates and infants up to the age of 4 months, depend on infant formula (and/or breast milk) to sustain their caloric and fluid needs. Therefore, calculation of caloric and fluid requirements is an integral part of pediatric medication dosage calculation. Additional fluid support for replacement therapy may be ordered to reverse fluid and electrolyte losses related to gastrointestinal disorders, such as vomiting, diarrhea, or fever.

Injectable and IV administration of medication dosages requires the use of a small-volume delivery system to prevent large-volume fluid overload, leading to toxicity. Calculating the drip rate is similar to the method used in calculating adult dosages, as presented in previous chapters, except the patient's BW or BSA needs to be factored into the DA setup.

A typical pediatric dosage calculation will include some, but not all, of the following:

1. The reference dose ordered (Ord)—all dosage orders
2. The available dosage (A)—all dosage orders
3. The patient's body weight (BW)—all dosage orders
4. The patient's body surface area (BSA)—orders with a reference dose using BSA
5. The schedule of doses ordered (Os)—all dosage orders
6. The drop factor (DF)—parenteral orders to monitor drip rate and flow rate
7. The flow time ordered (Oft)—intermittent parenteral orders.

If you have problems with lengthy setups that include drop factors (DF), reference doses (Ord), available doses (A), unit equivalency conversion factors (U), and the patient's body weight (BW) or body surface area (BSA), you can break the setup into two or three smaller units. If you decide to do this, be very careful not to make a mathematical mistake that you may carry from one setup to the next. Remember to make sure that all unwanted units cancel, and double-check the math.

PROBLEM SET	PROBLEM SET ANSWERS
1. Jamie, a 16-year-old patient, is receiving fluids intravenously. She tells you that she counted 20 drops of fluids entering the drip chamber every min, and she wants to know how much fluid she is receiving intravenously per d (use 15 gtt/ml).	1. 1920 ml/d

PROBLEM SET	PROBLEM SET ANSWERS

2. Heather received a new bag of 500 ml of D_5W at the beginning of your shift at 9:00 PM. The order was to administer 500 ml IV over 8 hr. Calculate the drip rate in gtt/min (15 gtt/ml), and the flow rate in ml/hr.

2. 15.6 gtt = 16 gtt/min
62.5 ml/hr

3. An aminophylline loading dose of 6 mg/kg in 100 ml of D_5W IVPB over 20 min was ordered for Timmy, who weighs 74 lb. Aminophylline is available in 250 mg/10-ml vial. Calculate the number of ml/dose.

3. 8.1 ml/dose

4. Zofran (ondansetron HCl) 20 mg in 50 cc of D_5W over 15 min was ordered prior to chemotherapy for prevention of gastrointestinal side effects. Calculate the drip rate using the microdrop factor, μgtt/min.

4. 200 μgtt/min

5. An insulin drip at 8 U/hr was ordered. Available is Humulin R 200 U in 500 ml of NS. Calculate the flow rate in ml/hr.

5. 20 ml/hr

6. Alprostadil 0.1 μg/kg per min continuous IV infusion was ordered for baby Bobby for temporary maintenance of patent ductus arteriosus while he is awaiting surgery. Alprostadil is available in 500 μg/250 ml of NS. Baby Bobby weighs 5 lb 6 oz. Calculate the drip rate in μgtt/min.

6. 7.3 = 7 μgtt/min

7. A Nembutal (pentobarbital) loading dose of 15 mg/kg in 500 ml of NS IV over 2 hr was ordered for Michael, a 16-year-old comatose teenager, who weighs 159 lb. Calculate the drip rate in gtt/min (15 gtt/ml).

7. 62.5 = 63 gtt/min

PROBLEM SET	PROBLEM SET ANSWERS
8. Intravenous administration of Nembutal should not exceed 50 mg/min. Is the rate of administration in Question 7 appropriate?	8. The rate of administration is 9 mg/min. It is appropriate.
9. Little Lucy weighs 27 lb, which is normal for her height. Convert her BW to BSA.	9. 0.55 m^2
10. The reference dose for Demerol is 1 mg/kg per dose. Meperidine HCl is available in 25 mg/ml. Your patient weighs 33 lb. Calculate the number of ml/dose.	10. 0.6 ml/dose
11. Phenobarbital 5 mg/kg SC qPM was ordered for Mickey, who weighs 46 lb. Phenobarbital is available in 130 mg/ml. Calculate the number of ml/dose.	11. 0.8 ml/dose
12. Filgrastim 10 μg/kg per d SC for 14 d is ordered for Nellie, who weighs 56 lb. Available is Neupogen 300 μg/ml. Calculate the number of ml/d.	12. 0.85 ml/d
13. The reference dose for Sus-Phrine (epinephrine) is 0.005 ml/kg per 15 min SC repeated 3 times p.r.n. Your patient weighs 78 lb. Calculate the number of ml/dose.	13. 0.18 ml/dose

PROBLEM SET	PROBLEM SET ANSWERS

14. Roferon-A (interferon alpha-2a [recombinant]) 2 mU/m^2 per d SC was ordered for Marcie, who weighs 60 lb and is 55 in. tall. Roferon-A is available in 6 mU/ml. What is her BSA? Calculate the number of ml/d.

    14. BSA = 1 m^2
        0.33 ml/d

15. The reference dose for morphine sulfate is 0.1 mg/kg per dose IM q4hr p.r.n. (max 15 mg/dose). Jeremiah weighs 94 lb. Morphine sulfate is available in 5 mg/ml Tubex cartridges. Calculate the number of ml/dose.

    15. 0.85 ml/dose

16. The reference dose for Sandostatin is 5 μg/kg per dose IVSP over 3 min q12hr (max 50 μg/dose). Your patient weighs 58 lb. Octreotide acetate is available in 0.1 mg/ml ampules. Calculate the number of ml/dose.

    16. 1.3 ml/dose

17. Hydrocortone 15 mg/m^2 per d IM q.d. is ordered for physiologic replacement therapy for little Markie, who weighs 14 lb (normal for his age and ht). Hydrocortisone is available in 25 mg/ml. What is his BSA? Calculate the number of ml/dose.

    17. a. 0.34 m^2
        b. 0.2 ml/dose

18. Jose, who is 7 years old, weighs 66 lb. Epinephrine (1 : 10,000) 0.01 mg/kg IV q5min was ordered to treat his sinus bradycardia. Calculate the number of mg/dose.

    18. 0.3 mg

19. For Cody's fever, the reference dose for Tylenol is 1 gr/y of age q.i.d. Cody is 3 years old. Tylenol elixir is available in 120 mg/tsp. Calculate the number of tsp/dose.

    19. 1½ tsp

PROBLEM SET	PROBLEM SET ANSWERS
20. Sally weighs 36 lb. Calculate Sally's minimum fluid requirement in ml/d.	20. 1318 ml/d
21. Digoxin is available in 50 μg/ml. The reference dose for digoxin is 8 μg/kg per dose. Joanie weighs 18.75 kg. Calculate the number of ml/dose.	21. 3 ml
22. The reference dose for pseudoephedrine for children is 4 mg/kg per d given q.i.d. Pseudoephedrine syrup comes in 15 mg/5 ml. Calculate the number of ml/dose for Cynthia, who weighs 28 lb.	22. 4.2 = 4 ml
23. The reference dose for Biaxin (clarithromycin) is 15 mg/kg per d PO given b.i.d. Calculate the number of tsp/dose for Dora, who weighs 37 lb. Biaxin suspension is available in 125 mg/tsp.	23. 1 tsp/dose
24. Sally is a 4-month-old infant, who weighs 14 lb 5 oz (140 to 150 kcal/kg per d). She is receiving Enfamil with Fe (40 kcal/fl oz). a. Calculate Sally's daily caloric needs. b. How many fl oz does she need to consume daily?	24. a. 910 to 975 kcal/d b. 23 to 24 fl oz/d
25. Molly weighs 11 lb. Calculate Molly's minimum fluid requirement in fl oz. The reference minimum fluid requirement for pediatric patients is: 100 ml/kg per d for the first 10 kg 50 ml/kg per d for the next 10 kg 20 ml/kg per d for each additional kg of BW	25. 16.7, that is, 16 to 17 fl oz/d

PROBLEM SET

26. The order to relieve Mary's pain is morphine sulfate 0.02 mg/kg per hr continuous IV infusion. Mary weighs 42 lb. Available is morphine sulfate 2 mg in 100 ml of NS. Calculate the drip rate in μgtt/min and the flow rate in ml/hr.

26. a. 19 μgtt/min
    b. 19 ml/hr

27. Intropin 3 μg/kg per min continuous IV infusion was ordered to increase the renal blood flow of Lacey, who weighs 25 lb. Available is dopamine HCl 40 mg/500 ml of NS. Calculate the flow rate in ml/hr.

27. 25.57 = 26 ml/hr

28. Continuous IV infusion of heparin at 15 U/kg per hr was ordered for Letasha, who weighs 39 lb. Heparin sodium is available in 1000 U/250 ml. Calculate the drip rate in μgtt/min.

28. 66.47 = 66 μgtt/min

29. Inocor 5 μg/kg per min was ordered for Susie, who weighs 57 lb. Amrinone lactate is available in 50 mg/250 ml of NS. Calculate the flow rate in ml/hr.

29. 38.86 = 39 ml/hr

30. Solu-Medrol 20 mg/m^2 per d IM b.i.d. was ordered for Jessica, who weighs 49 lb (normal wt for ht). Methylprednisolone sodium succinate is available in 125 mg reconstituted to a total volume of 8 ml in a single-dose Act-O-Vial system.

a. What is Jessica's BSA?
b. Calculate the number of ml/dose

30. a. 0.858 m^2
    b. 0.55 ml/dose

In the following examples, DA will be applied to calculate medication dosage.

Educate and inform the patient and obtain her signature on the consent form prior to administration.

A × O = Ans

This is just another PO medication order. If you are still not sure how to set up the DA process, there are numerous examples in Chapter 4 for you to review.

A × O = Ans

A × O = Ans

Provide the patient with educational material on sexually transmitted diseases (STD).

E X A M P L E   1

Marcie opted for an injectable form of contraceptive. The provider ordered Depo-Provera 150 mg IM q3mo. Available is medroxyprogesterone acetate 100 mg/ml in a 5-ml vial. Calculate the number of ml/dose.

Pertinent information provided: 150 mg/dose; 100 mg/ml
Unit equivalency conversion: None needed
Desired unit: ml/dose

CORRECT setup:

$$\frac{ml}{100\ mg} \times \frac{150\ mg}{dose} = 1.5\ ml/dose$$

E X A M P L E   2

Genie and Lloyd are trying to start a family. After a consultation, the provider ordered Provera (medroxyprogesterone acetate) 10 mg PO for 5 days to induce withdrawal bleeding. Provera is available in 10-mg tab. Calculate the number of tab/dose.

Pertinent information provided: 10 mg/dose; 10-mg tab
Unit equivalency conversion: None needed
Desired unit: tab/dose

CORRECT setup:

$$\frac{tab}{10\ mg} \times \frac{10\ mg}{dose} = 1\ tab$$

E X A M P L E   3

On the first day of withdrawal bleeding, Clomid 50 mg PO q.d. is ordered for Genie. Clomid is available in 50-mg tab. Calculate the number of tab/dose.

Pertinent information provided: 50 mg/dose; 50-mg tab
Unit equivalency conversion: None needed
Desired unit: tab/dose

CORRECT setup:

$$\frac{tab}{50\ mg} \times \frac{50\ mg}{dose} = 1\ tab$$

E X A M P L E   4

Zithromax 1 gm PO single dose stat for treatment of *Chlamydia trachomatis* is ordered for a patient. Available is azithromycin 250-mg tab. Calculate the number of tab/dose.

Pertinent information provided: 1 gm/dose; 250-mg tab
Unit equivalency conversion: 1000 mg/gm
Desired unit: tab/dose

CORRECT setup:

$$\frac{\text{tab}}{250 \text{ mg}} \times \frac{1 \text{ gm}}{\text{dose}} \times \frac{1000 \text{ mg}}{\text{gm}} = 4 \text{ tab/dose}$$

A × O × U = Ans

E X A M P L E   5

An iron supplement was ordered for Linda. The order reads $FeSO_4$ 5 gr PO b.i.d. Available is $FeSO_4$ 325-mg tab. Calculate the number of mg/d.
  Pertinent information provided: 5 gr/dose; 2 dose/d
  Unit equivalency conversion: 60 to 65 mg/gr
  Desired unit: mg/d

CORRECT setup:

$$\frac{2 \text{ dose}}{\text{d}} \times \frac{5 \text{ gr}}{\text{dose}} \times \frac{60 \text{ to } 65 \text{ mg}}{\text{gr}} = 600 \text{ to } 650 \text{ mg/d}$$

Read the question carefully.

Os = b.i.d. = 2 dose/d

Os × O × U = Ans

M I N I   Q U I Z

How many tab/d will Linda need?

Answer: 2 tab/d

If you use 60 mg/gr, the tab/dose will be 1.8 tab/dose. If you use 65 mg/gr, the tab/dose will be exactly 2 tab/dose. In either case, you will round your answer to the nearest measurable unit dose of 2 tab/dose.

Round your answers to the nearest measurable unit.

E X A M P L E   6

RhoGAM 300 μg IM stat is ordered for Marianne, who tested Rh negative at week 40 of gestation. Available is a RhoGAM 300-μg, single-dose syringe. What will you need to do to carry out this order?

- Complete the patient identification cards and the necessary forms. RhoGAM is stored under refrigeration.
- To administer, warm the single-dose syringe containing RhoGAM 300 μg.
- Administer an IM injection, taking care not to deliver the medication into the circulatory system.

RhoGAM requires a storage temperature of 2 to 8°C.

Check the refrigerator and freezer for accuracy with a thermometer and keep a daily temperature log. Improper storage changes the therapeutic effects of medications.

Aspirate the needle prior to injection.

E X A M P L E   7

An order to treat Darlene's threatened abortion is lactated Ringer's solution at 200 ml/hr, bed rest, and sexual abstinence. Calculate the IV rate in gtt/min (15 gtt/ml).
  Pertinent information provided: 200 ml/hr; 15 gtt/ml
  Unit equivalency conversion: 60 min/hr
  Desired unit: gtt/min

CORRECT setup:

$$\frac{15 \text{ gtt}}{\text{ml}} \times \frac{200 \text{ ml}}{\text{hr}} \times \frac{\text{hr}}{60 \text{ min}} = 50 \text{ gtt/min}$$

Threatened Abortion. Involves a gestation of less than 20 wk with uterine bleeding, but without cervical dilation or expulsion of tissue.

DF = 15 gtt/ml
Or = 200 ml/hr

DF × Or × U = Ans

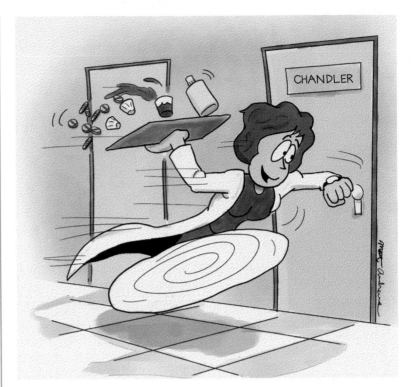

"9:28, 9:29, 9:30 ... NOW I CAN GIVE
MRS. CHANDLER HER 10:00 MEDS!"

Calculations for Administration of Antepartum Medications

The following examples represent common fluid and medication orders given for antepartum complications.

 You will need to follow the established toxic chemical protocol to handle, dispense, and dispose of methotrexate.

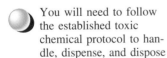 Use the BW, ht, and BSA nomogram to determine that the patient's BSA = 1.7 m².

 Ord = 50 mg/m²/dose.

 A × Ord × BSA = Ans

E X A M P L E   1

A single dose of methotrexate 50 mg/m² IM is ordered to treat an ectopic gestation. Gail weighs 138 lb and measures 64 inches tall. Available is methotrexate sodium 100 mg/4 ml. Calculate the number of ml/dose.

Pertinent information provided: 50 mg/m² per dose; 138 lb, 64 in.; 100 mg/4 ml

Unit equivalency conversion: From nomogram (see Appendix)

Desired unit: ml/dose

CORRECT setup:

$$\frac{4 \text{ ml}}{100 \text{ mg}} \times \frac{50 \text{ mg}}{\text{m}^2 \cdot \text{dose}} \times 1.7 \text{ m}^2 = 3.4 \text{ ml/dose}$$

Because 3.4 ml is too large to administer in a single dose, you will need to administer it in two divided doses.

E X A M P L E   2

Tigan 200-mg suppository PR t.i.d. was ordered to treat Susan's hyperemesis gravidarum. Available are trimethobenzamide HCl 100-mg suppositories. Calculate the number of supp/dose.

Pertinent information provided: 200 mg/dose; 100-mg supp
Unit equivalency conversion: None needed
Desired unit: supp/dose

CORRECT setup:

$$\frac{supp}{100 \text{ mg}} \times \frac{200 \text{ mg}}{dose} = 2 \text{ supp/dose}$$

 Apply gentle pressure against the anal sphincter for a few seconds to relax the muscle for easy insertion of the suppository. Apply a water-based lubricant, if appropriate, for added comfort.

 A × O = Ans

E X A M P L E   3

Karen has no health insurance. She is ordered nitrofurantoin monohydrate 100 mg PO b.i.d. for 10 d for her urinary tract infection. Available is a sample medication of Macrobid 100-mg capsule (cap). Calculate the number of cap/10 d she will need.

Pertinent information provided: 2 dose/d; 1 cap/dose; 10 d
Unit equivalency conversion: None needed
Desired unit: cap/10 d

CORRECT setup:

$$\frac{1 \text{ cap}}{dose} \times \frac{2 \text{ dose}}{d} \times 10 \text{ d} = 20 \text{ cap/10 d}$$

 Pharmaceutical companies frequently provide samples to providers for treatment.

 Os = 2 dose/d; Ot = 10 d

 O × Os × Ot = Ans

E X A M P L E   4

Celestone phosphate 12 mg IM q.d. × 2 doses was ordered for Nadine. Available is betamethasone sodium phosphate 20 mg/ml. Calculate the number of ml/dose.

Pertinent information provided: 12 mg/dose; 20 mg/ml
Unit equivalency conversion: None needed
Desired unit: ml/dose

CORRECT setup:

$$\frac{ml}{20 \text{ mg}} \times \frac{12 \text{ mg}}{dose} = 0.6 \text{ ml/dose}$$

 If you do not know the generic and trade names for medications, look them up in a drug reference book.

 A × O = Ans

E X A M P L E   5

Ampicillin 2 gm IVPB over 60 min q6hr is ordered, to treat pyelonephritis. Available is ampicillin sodium 2 gm/100 ml NS. Calculate the flow rate in ml/hr.

 Inspect all parenteral products for particulation and discoloration prior to administration. Do not use a discolored product or one that contains a particulate.

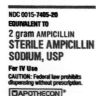

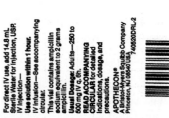

Or = dose/time =
2 gm/60 min

A × Or × U = Ans

Or = 40 mg/hr;
A = 200 mg/500 ml

A × Or = Ans

The problem provides far more information than you need to solve what it is asking you to do. Be sure to sift out the pertinent information to solve this problem.

DF = 10 gtt/ml;
Or = Ov/Ot =
250 ml/20 min

DF × Or = Ans

DF × Ov × Ot = Ans

A = 25,000 U/250 ml;
Ord = 15 U/kg/h; BW = 189 lb

Round fractions to the nearest ml, because most volume infusion pumps do not allow entry of decimal fractions.

A × Ord × U × BW = Ans

Pertinent information provided: 2 gm/60 min; 2 gm/100 ml
Unit equivalency conversion: None needed
Desired unit: ml/hr

CORRECT setup:

$$\frac{100 \text{ ml}}{2 \text{ gm}} \times \frac{2 \text{ gm}}{60 \text{ min}} \times \frac{60 \text{ min}}{hr} = 100 \text{ ml/hr}$$

E X A M P L E   6

Trandate 40 mg/hr IV over 30 min was ordered for Eugenia, who is experiencing preeclamptic hypertension. Available is labetalol HCl 200 mg in 500 ml D$_5$W. Calculate the flow rate in ml/hr.
   Pertinent information provided: 40 mg/hr; 200 mg/500 ml
   Unit equivalency conversion: None needed
   Desired unit: ml/hr

CORRECT setup:

$$\frac{500 \text{ ml}}{200 \text{ mg}} \times \frac{40 \text{ mg}}{hr} = 100 \text{ ml/hr}$$

E X A M P L E   7

An aminophylline loading dose of 5 mg/kg in 250 ml D$_5$W IV over 20 min is ordered for Margaret's acute asthmatic exacerbation. Margaret is 6 mo pregnant and weighs 148 lb. Calculate the drip rate in gtt/min (10 gtt/ml).
   Pertinent information provided: 250 ml/20 min; 10 gtt/ml
   Unit equivalency conversion: None needed
   Desired unit: gtt/min

CORRECT setup:

$$\frac{10 \text{ gtt}}{ml} \times \frac{250 \text{ ml}}{20 \text{ min}} = 125 \text{ gtt/min}$$

or

$$\frac{10 \text{ gtt}}{ml} \times \frac{250 \text{ ml}}{dose} \times \frac{dose}{20 \text{ min}} = 125 \text{ gtt/min}$$

E X A M P L E   8

Heparin 15 U/kg per hr IV is ordered to treat Grace's deep-vein thrombosis, experienced at 24 wk gestation. Grace weighs 189 lb. Available is heparin 25,000 U in 250 ml D$_5$W. Calculate the flow rate in ml/hr.
   Pertinent information provided: 15 U/kg per hr; 189 lb; 25,000 U/250 ml
   Unit equivalency conversion: 2.2 lb/kg
   Desired unit: ml/hr

CORRECT setup:

$$\frac{250 \text{ ml}}{25,000 \text{ U}} \times \frac{15 \text{ U}}{kg \cdot hr} \times \frac{kg}{2.2 \text{ lb}} \times 189 \text{ lb} = 12.9 = 13 \text{ ml/hr}$$

EXAMPLE 9

To manage Irene's diabetes, Humulin R* 1.5 U/hr IVPB with ½ NS to KVO is ordered. Available is Humulin R 40 U in 500 ml of NS. Calculate the number of μgtt/min.

Pertinent information provided: 1.5 U/hr; 40 U/500 ml
Unit equivalency conversion: 60 min/hr; 60 μgtt/ml
Desired unit: μgtt/min

CORRECT setup:

$$\frac{60 \; \mu gtt}{ml} \times \frac{500 \; ml}{40 \; U} \times \frac{1.5 \; U}{hr} \times \frac{hr}{60 \; min} = 18.75 = 19 \; \mu gtt/min$$

Or = 1.5 U/hr

DF × A × Or × U = Ans

MINI QUIZ

Can you convert the drip rate between μgtt and gtt?

Answer: Yes

DF of 15 gtt/ml = 60 divided by 4
DF of 10 gtt/ml = 60 divided by 6

Calculations for Administration of Medications During Labor and Delivery

The following are examples of medication dosage calculations for administration of medications during labor and delivery.

EXAMPLE 1

Prepidil gel (dinoprostone 0.5 mg/gel) ¹⁄₁₂₀ gr PV q6hr, 2 doses, is ordered for cervical priming in a post-term pregnancy. Available is dinoprostone 0.5 mg/2.5 ml in a single-dose syringe applicator. Calculate the number of applicator (appl)/dose.

Pertinent information provided: ¹⁄₁₂₀ gr/dose; 0.5 mg/appl
Unit equivalency conversion: 60 mg/gr
Desired unit: appl/dose

CORRECT setup:

$$\frac{1 \; appl}{0.5 \; mg} \times \frac{1 \; gr}{120 \; dose} \times \frac{60 \; mg}{gr} = 1 \; appl/dose$$

Wear gloves to avoid skin contact.

Warm Prepidil to room temperature for administration.

A × O × U = Ans

EXAMPLE 2

Jocelyn went into premature labor at 33 wk of gestation. Along with bed rest in the left lateral decubitus position, LR 1 L at 150 ml/hr was ordered. Calculate the number of hr before you hang the next bag of 1 L lactated Ringer's solution (LR).

Pertinent information provided: 150 ml/hr; 1 L
Unit equivalency conversion: 1000 ml/L
Desired unit: hr/L

CORRECT setup:

$$\frac{hr}{150 \; ml} \times \frac{1000 \; ml}{L} = 6.67 \; hr/L = 6 \; hr \; 40 \; min$$

Premature Labor. Occurs when labor commences after week 20 but before week 37 of gestation.

Or = 150 ml/hr

Or × U = Ans

---

*Humulin® R is a registered trademark of Eli Lilly and Company.

Review the nursing diag-
noses that accompany
each medication in your
drug manual before you
administer the medication
dosage.

A × U × O = Ans

% solution = gm/100 ml
50% = 50 gm/100 ml

A × O = Ans

Oxytocin is a uterine
stimulant for induction of
labor.

A × O = Ans

A × O = Ans

EXAMPLE   3

Jocelyn's fetal pulse rate decreased below 110 beats/min, so the provider
ordered terbutaline 250 μg SQ q2hr × 2 doses. Available is terbutaline sul-
fate 1 mg/ml. Calculate the number of ml/dose.
  Pertinent information provided: 250 μg/dose; 1 mg/ml
  Unit equivalency conversion: 1000 μg/mg
  Desired unit: ml/dose

CORRECT setup:

$$\frac{\text{ml}}{1 \ \cancel{\text{mg}}} \times \frac{\cancel{\text{mg}}}{1000 \ \cancel{\mu g}} \times \frac{250 \ \cancel{\mu g}}{\text{dose}} = 0.25 \ \text{ml/dose}$$

EXAMPLE   4

During labor, Lorraine started to seize. Magnesium sulfate 4 gm IVSP over
5 min stat is ordered. Available is magnesium sulfate 50% 2-ml vial. Calcu-
late the number of ml/dose.
  Pertinent information provided: 4 gm/dose; 50% = 50 gm/100 ml
  Unit equivalency conversion: None needed
  Desired unit: ml/dose

CORRECT setup:

$$\frac{100 \ \text{ml}}{50 \ \cancel{\text{gm}}} \times \frac{4 \ \cancel{\text{gm}}}{\text{dose}} = 8 \ \text{ml/dose}$$

EXAMPLE   5

You need to prepare oxytocin 40 U in LR 1 L on standby in case of
postpartum hemorrhage. Oxytocin is available in 10 U/ml. Calculate the
number of ml you will need to inject into the LR 1-L solution.
  Pertinent information provided: 40 U/dose; 10 U/ml
  Unit equivalency conversion: None needed
  Desired unit: ml/dose

CORRECT setup:

$$\frac{\text{ml}}{10 \ \cancel{\text{U}}} \times \frac{40 \ \cancel{\text{U}}}{\text{dose}} = 4 \ \text{ml/dose}$$

EXAMPLE   6

In addition to magnesium sulfate, pentobarbital 125 mg IVSP over 3 min is
ordered. Available is Nembutal 50 mg/ml. Calculate the number of ml/dose.
  Pertinent information provided: 125 mg/dose; 50 mg/ml
  Unit equivalency conversion: None needed
  Desired unit: ml/dose

CORRECT setup:

$$\frac{\text{ml}}{50 \ \cancel{\text{mg}}} \times \frac{125 \ \cancel{\text{mg}}}{\text{dose}} = 2.5 \ \text{ml/dose}$$

E X A M P L E   7

Isabella went into premature labor at 34 wk of gestation. Yutopar, 50 μg/min for 20 min and then increased to 100 μg/min, is ordered. Available is ritodrine HCl 150 mg in 500 ml of D_5NS. Calculate the flow rate in ml/hr for the first 20 min and thereafter.

   Pertinent information provided: 50 μg/min; 180 μg/min; 150 mg/500 ml

   Unit equivalency conversion: 60 min/hr; 1000 μg/mg

   Desired unit: ml/hr

CORRECT setup:

1. The first 20 min at 50 μg/min

$$\frac{500 \text{ ml}}{150 \text{ mg}} \times \frac{\text{mg}}{1000 \text{ } \mu g} \times \frac{50 \text{ } \mu g}{\text{min}} \times \frac{60 \text{ min}}{\text{hr}} = 10 \text{ ml/hr}$$

2. Thereafter at 100 μg/min

$$\frac{500 \text{ ml}}{150 \text{ mg}} \times \frac{\text{mg}}{1000 \text{ } \mu g} \times \frac{100 \text{ } \mu g}{\text{min}} \times \frac{60 \text{ min}}{\text{hr}} = 20 \text{ ml/hr}$$

Ritodrine is a uterine re-laxant for arresting pre-mature labor.

Or = 50 μg/min
    = 100 μg/min

A $\times$ U $\times$ Or $\times$ U = Ans

A $\times$ U $\times$ Or $\times$ U = Ans

E X A M P L E   8

To induce labor, Pitocin is ordered as follows: 0.5 mU (milliunit)/min IV. Increase by doubling the dose q30min until there are three contractions every 10 min. Available is oxytocin 10 U in 1 L of D_5W. Calculate the flow rate in ml/hr.

   Pertinent information provided: 0.5 mU/min; 10 U/L

   Unit equivalency conversion: 1000 mU/U; 1000 ml/L

   Desired unit: ml/hr

CORRECT setup:

$$\frac{1000 \text{ ml}}{\text{L}} \times \frac{\text{L}}{10 \text{ U}} \times \frac{\text{U}}{1000 \text{ mU}} \times \frac{0.5 \text{ mU}}{\text{min}} \times \frac{60 \text{ min}}{\text{hr}} = 3 \text{ ml/hr}$$
$$\quad \text{U} \quad \times \quad \text{A} \quad \times \quad \text{U} \quad \times \quad \text{Or} \quad \times \quad \text{U} \quad = \quad \text{Ans}$$

1000 mU = 1 unit; that is, 1000 mU = 1 U

M I N I   Q U I Z

Calculate the number of gtt/min after 2hr of Pitocin induction.

Answer: Flow rate doubled at 30 min, 60 min, 90 min, and 120 min (2 hr) = 48 ml/hr

Calculations for Administration of Postpartum Medications

The following are examples of dosage calculations for the administration of common medication orders for the postpartum population.

Check all unit dimensions and do the necessary unit equivalency conversion(s).

Joanne complained of breast tenderness and soon developed postpartum mastitis. Dicloxacillin 2 gm/d PO q.i.d. is ordered. Available is dicloxacillin 500-mg tab. Calculate the number of tab/dose.

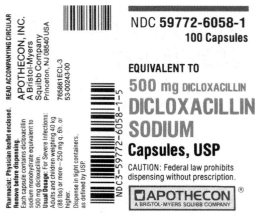

Pertinent information provided: 2 gm/d; 4 dose/d; 500 mg/tab
Unit equivalency conversion: 1000 mg/gm
Desired unit: tab/dose

 Os = q.i.d. = 4 dose/d;
Or = 2 gm/d

CORRECT setup:

$$\frac{tab}{500\ mg} \times \frac{1000\ mg}{gm} \times \frac{2\ gm}{d} \times \frac{d}{4\ dose} = 1\ tab/dose$$

 A × U × Or × Os = Ans

Methergine 0.2 mg IM stat is ordered to control postpartum hemorrhage. Available is methergine 0.2 mg/ml. Calculate the number of ml/dose of methergine.
Pertinent information provided: 0.2 mg/dose; 0.2 mg/ml
Unit equivalency conversion: None needed
Desired unit: ml/dose

 A × O = Ans

CORRECT setup:

$$\frac{ml}{0.2\ mg} \times \frac{0.2\ mg}{dose} = 1\ ml/dose$$

$FeSO_4$ 16¼ gr/d PO t.i.d. is ordered for Rolinda's postpartum anemia. Available is $FeSO_4$ 325 mg tab. Calculate the number of tab/dose.

Pertinent information provided: 16¼ = ⁶⁵⁄₄ gr/d; 3 dose/d; 325 mg/tab
Unit equivalency conversion: 60 mg/gr
Desired unit: tab/dose

 Or = 16¼ gr/d;
Os = t.i.d. = 3 dose/d

CORRECT setup:

$$\frac{tab}{325 \; \cancel{mg}} \times \frac{60 \; \cancel{mg}}{\cancel{gr}} \times \frac{65 \; \cancel{gr}}{4 \; \cancel{d}} \times \frac{\cancel{d}}{3 \; dose} = 1 \; tab/dose$$

Notice the orientation of the dimension (gr/d) linked to 16¼ remains the same, that is,

$$16\tfrac{1}{4} = 65/4 \; gr/d = \frac{65 \; gr}{4 \; d}$$

Convert the mixed number to a fraction, that is, $16\tfrac{1}{4} = {}^{65}\!/_{4}$

A × U × Or × Os = Ans

E X A M P L E   4

To improve $FeSO_4$ absorption, vitamin C 250 mg PO t.i.d. is ordered. Available is vitamin C 500-mg chewable tab. Calculate the number of tab/dose.
   Pertinent information provided: 250 mg/dose; 500 mg/tab
   Unit equivalency conversion: None needed
   Desired unit: tab/dose

CORRECT setup:

$$\frac{tab}{500 \; \cancel{mg}} \times \frac{250 \; \cancel{mg}}{dose} = \tfrac{1}{2} \; tab/dose$$

A × O = Ans

E X A M P L E   5a

Gentamicin 2 mg/kg IVPB now (max 120 mg/dose) is ordered for treatment of postpartum endomyometritis. Marilyn weighs 145 lb. Available is gentamicin sulfate in vials of 40 mg/ml and 100 mg/ml.
Calculate the number of mg/dose.
   Pertinent information provided: 2 mg/kg; 145 lb; max: 120 mg/dose
   Unit equivalency conversion: 2.2 lb/kg
   Desired unit: mg/dose

CORRECT setup:

$$\frac{2 \; mg}{\cancel{kg}} \times \frac{\cancel{kg}}{2.2 \; \cancel{lb}} \times 145 \; \cancel{lb} = 132 \; mg/dose$$

The answer is 120 mg/dose, because 132 mg/dose exceeds the maximum allowable dosage of 120 mg/dose.

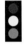

A medication dosage cannot go above or below the reference dose range, that is, the minimum and maximum allowable amounts of medication per dose or d.

Ord = 2 mg/kg

Ord × U × BW = Ans

E X A M P L E   5b

To continue treatment of Marilyn's (BW = 145 lb) postpartum endomyometritis, gentamicin 1.5 mg/kg IVPB q8hr is ordered. You have in stock D_5W 50 ml and gentamicin sulfate in vials of 40 mg/ml and 100 mg/ml.

1. Calculate the number of mg/dose.
2. Which available form of gentamicin sulfate will you use?
3. Calculate the number of ml/dose of gentamicin sulfate.

   Pertinent information provided: 1.5 mg/kg; 145 lb; 40 mg/ml and/or 100 mg/ml
   Unit equivalency conversion: None needed
   Desired unit: mg/dose

To avoid medication wastage, choose the available dosage form closest to your need.

Ord = 1.5 mg/kg

If you chose the gentami-
cin sulfate vial of 40 mg/
ml, you would have had
to use three vials, or 120
mg of medication,
whereas you need only
99 mg. You would have
wasted a lot of medica-
tion unnecessarily.

Ord × U × BW = Ans

O × A = Ans

CORRECT setup:

$$\frac{1.5 \text{ mg}}{\cancel{\text{kg}}} \times \frac{\cancel{\text{kg}}}{2.2 \cancel{\text{lb}}} \times 145 \cancel{\text{lb}} = 99 \text{ mg/dose}$$

The form of gentamicin sulfate available as 100 mg/ml will be preferable over the 40-mg/ml vial.

$$\frac{99 \cancel{\text{mg}}}{\text{dose}} \times \frac{\text{ml}}{100 \cancel{\text{mg}}} = 0.99 \text{ ml} = 1 \text{ ml/dose}$$

Chapter Summary

This chapter has demonstrated some common dosages of fluid and medication orders given to the obstetric population. The scenarios presented were realistic. Obstetric orders include all forms of topical, oral, injectable, and parenteral dosages. Moreover, orders can be based on the reference dose, depending on the medication. Therefore, you will need to include the conversion factors pertaining to BW, (for example, mg/kg), BSA, (for example, mg/m²), and dosage rate (for example, mg/kg per hr). Use of DA in calculating dosages frees you from the task of remembering mathematical and algebraic formulas.

If you are still having difficulty with the process of DA, it is important that you go back to Chapters 3, 4, and 5 and review the examples presented. An integral part of the learning process involves exercising the new skills learned. With continuing practice and use, you will master the process!

PROBLEM SET	PROBLEM SET ANSWERS
1. Ordered: Nubain 5 mg SQ q2hr Available: Vial of nalbuphine HCl 20 mg/ml Calculate the number of ml/dose.	1. 0.25 ml/dose
2. Ordered: Demerol 100 mg IM q4hr Available: Single-dose syringe of meperidine 100 mg/ml Calculate the number of ml/dose.	2. 1 ml/dose

PROBLEM	PROBLEM SET	PROBLEM SET ANSWERS

PROBLEM

13. You need
correct d
94 ml/hr.

14. Ordered:
Calculate

15. Ordered:
Available
Calculate

16. Ordered:
Available
Calculate

17. Ordered:
Available:
Calculate

PROBLEM SET

3. Ordered: Phenergan 25 mg IM p.r.n.
Available: Multidose vial of promethazine 500 mg/10 ml
Calculate the number of ml/dose.

4. Ordered: Stadol 2 mg IM q4hr
Available: Butorphanol tartrate 1 mg/ml
Calculate the number of ml/dose.

5. Ordered: D_5LR (dextrose in lactated Ringer's solution) at 125 ml/hr
Calculate the drip rate in gtt/min (10 gtt/ml).

6. Ordered: Fleet saline enema PR now
Available: Fleet saline enema, 4½ fl oz, ready-to-use squeeze bottle
Calculate the number of ml/dose.

7. Ordered: Narcan 0.4 mg IM now
Available: Naloxone HCl 0.4 mg/ml
Calculate the number of ml/dose.

PROBLEM SET ANSWERS

3. 0.5 ml/dose

4. 2 ml/dose

5. $20.8 = 21$ gtt/min

6. 135 ml/dose

7. 1 ml/dose

PROBL

PROBLEM SET

8. Ord
   Ava
   Cal
   a. a
   b. c

18. Ordered: D$_5$LR with 20 mEq KCl (potassium chloride) 1 L at 150 ml/hr
    Available: D$_5$LR 1 L bag and KCl 40 mEq/20-ml vial
    a. Calculate the number ml of KCl/1 L D$_5$LR.
    b. Calculate the drip rate in gtt/min (15 gtt/ml).
    c. Calculate the number of hr/L.

18. a. 10 ml KCl/1 L
       D$_5$LR
    b. 37.5 = 38 gtt/min
    c. 6 hr 40 min

9. Orde
   Ava
   Calc

19. Ordered: Heparin 5000 U at 1200 U/hr
    Available: Heparin 5000 U in 100 ml D$_5$W
    Calculate the flow rate in ml/hr.

19. 24 ml/hr

10. Orde
    Avai
    Calcu

20. Ordered: RhoGAM 50 μg IM now
    Available: RhoGAM 300 μg/ml single-dose syringe
    Calculate the number of ml/dose.

20. 0.17 ml/dose

11. Order
    Avail
    a. Ca
    b. Ca

21. Ordered: Oxytocin 10 U in D$_5$LR 1 L at 1 mU/min
    Available: Oxytocin 10 U/ml single-dose Tubex cartridge
    a. Calculate the number of ml/L D$_5$LR.
    b. Calculate the flow rate in ml/hr.
    c. Calculate the drip rate in μgtt/min.

21. a. 1 ml/L D$_5$LR
    b. 6 ml/h
    c. 6 μgtt/min

12. Ordere
    Availa
    Calcul

PROBLEM SET | PROBLEM SET ANSWERS

22. Ordered: Heparin 5000 mg IV bolus followed by heparin 25,000 U continuous IV infusion at 1000 U/hr
Available: Heparin 10,000 U/ml vial and D_5W 250-ml unit bag
a. Calculate the number of ml of heparin for the bolus dose.
b. Calculate the number of ml of heparin you will need to inject into the D_5W 250-ml unit bag for continuous IV infusion.
c. Calculate the flow rate in ml/hr that reflects 1000 U/hr.
d. Calculate the total infusion time to administer 25,000 U of heparin.

22. a. ½ ml Heparin for bolus dose
b. 2.5 ml heparin for D_5W 250-ml unit bag
c. 10 ml/hr continuous infusion
d. 25 hr of infusion time

23. Ordered: Humulin R 0.5 U/hr continuous IV infusion
Available: Humulin R 25 U in 250 ml of NS
a. Calculate the flow rate in ml/hr.
b. Calculate the drip rate in μgtt/min.

23. a. 5 ml/hr
b. 5 μgtt/min

24. Ordered: Ritodrine 50 μg/min and then increase dosage by 50 μg/min q20min (max 350 μg/min) until labor stops
Available: Yutopar 100 mg in 1 L D_5NS (dextrose in normal saline)
a. Calculate the initial flow rate in ml/hr.
b. Calculate the flow rate after 60 min.
c. Calculate the flow rate at the maximum dosage of 350 μg/min.

24. a. 30 ml/hr initial dosage
b. 120 ml/hr after 60 min
c. 210 ml/hr maximum rate

25. Ordered: From the maximum dosage of Ritodrine 350 μg/min, decrease dosage by 50 μg/min qhr to a minimum of 100 μg/min
Available: Yutopar 100 mg in 1 L of D_5NS
Calculate the number of hr needed to reach minimum dosage rate.

25. It will take 5 hr to decrease dosage to 100 μg/min.

PROBLEM SET	PROBLEM SET ANSWERS
26. Ordered: Magnesium sulfate 4 gm over 20 min followed by 2 gm/hr continuous IV infusion Available: Magnesium sulfate 40 gm in 1 L of D_5NS a. Calculate the flow rate in ml/hr for the first 20 min. b. Calculate the flow rate equivalent to 2 gm/hr.	26. a. 300 ml/hr for 20 min b. 50 ml/hr continuous IV
27. Ordered: Aztreonam 3 gm IVPB over 30 min q8hr Available: Azactam in vials of 1 gm and 2 gm and D_5W 100-ml unit bags a. What will be an appropriate dosage form of Azactam to use? b. Calculate the number of gtt/min (15 gtt/ml).	27. One each of the 1-gm and 2-gm vials. At a higher cost, you can use three vials of the 1-gm dosage form. b. 50 gtt/min
28. Ordered: Timentin 3.1 gm IVPB over 15 min q6hr Available: Ticarcillin/clavulanate 3.1-gm (3 gm of ticarcillin, 0.1 gm of clavulanic acid) vial and D_5W 50-ml unit bag Calculate the drip rate in gtt/min (10 gtt/ml).	28. 33.3 = 33gtt/min
29. Ordered: Clindamycin HCl 900 mg IVSP q8hr Available: Cleocin 150 mg/ml in 2-, 4-, and 6-ml vial dosage forms What is your choice of Cleocin dosage form for this order?	29. The 6-ml vial

PROBLEM SET	PROBLEM SET ANSWERS

30. Ordered: Dicloxacillin 500 mg PO q6hr
    Available: Dicloxacillin 62.5 mg/tsp suspension, and 125-mg, 250-mg, 500-mg cap
    The patient, Margaret, has a sore throat and cannot swallow the pill form. Calculate the number of tsp/dose of suspension.

30.   8 tsp/dose

Do the three checks, review the five rights, and apply the nursing process in dosage administration.

 The primary goal of psychiatric nursing is to prevent patients from harming themselves or others.

Ord = 150 mg/d
Os = 3 dose/d
A = 25 mg/tab

 A × Ord × Os = Ans

 Do not crush a medication that has a timed-release mechanism, for example, the dosage forms of ER, SR, XL.

 U × A × O × Os = Ans

 Look up side effects and adverse reactions of medications to incorporate this information into the nursing process.

CALCULATIONS FOR ADMINISTRATION OF ANTIDEPRESSANT MEDICATIONS

Antidepressants are categorized as follows:

- Tricyclic agents (TCA)
- Monoamine oxidase inhibitors (MAO)
- Selective serotonin reuptake inhibitors (SSRI)
- Tetracyclic agents and derivatives of other chemical classes

The following examples demonstrate commonly ordered antidepressive agents, grouped according to the preceding classes.

Tricyclic Agents

E X A M P L E   1

Ordered: Elavil 150 mg/d PO t.i.d.
Available: Amitriptyline HCl 25-mg tab

Calculate the number of tab/dose.
Pertinent information provided: 150 mg/d; 3 dose/d; 25 mg/tab
Unit equivalency conversion: None needed
Desired unit: tab/dose

CORRECT setup:

$$\frac{\text{tab}}{25\ \cancel{\text{mg}}} \times \frac{150\ \cancel{\text{mg}}}{\cancel{\text{d}}} \times \frac{\cancel{\text{d}}}{3\ \text{dose}} = 2\ \text{tab/dose}$$

E X A M P L E   2

Ordered: Pamelor 30 mg/d PO t.i.d.
Available: Nortriptyline HCl 10 mg/5ml

Calculate the number of tsp/dose.
Pertinent information provided: 30 mg/d; 3 dose/d; 10 mg/5 ml
Unit equivalency conversion: 5 ml/tsp
Desired unit: tsp/dose

CORRECT setup:

$$\frac{\text{tsp}}{5\ \cancel{\text{ml}}} \times \frac{5\ \cancel{\text{ml}}}{10\ \cancel{\text{mg}}} \times \frac{30\ \cancel{\text{mg}}}{\cancel{\text{d}}} \times \frac{\cancel{\text{d}}}{3\ \text{dose}} = 1\ \text{tsp/dose}$$

Monoamine Oxidase Inhibitors

E X A M P L E   3

Ordered: Nardil ¼ gr PO b.i.d.
Available: Phenelzine sulfate 15-mg tab

Calculate the number of tab/dose.
Pertinent information provided: ¼ gr/dose; 15 mg/tab
Unit equivalency conversion: 60 mg/gr
Desired unit: tab/dose

CORRECT setup:

$$\frac{tab}{15\ mg} \times \frac{60\ mg}{gr} \times \frac{1\ gr}{4\ dose} = 1\ tab/dose$$

60 to 65 mg = 1 gr
A × U × O = Ans

EXAMPLE 4

Ordered: Parnate ½ gr/d PO t.i.d.
Available: Tranylcypromine sulfate 10-mg tab

Calculate the number of tab/dose.

Look up the contraindications of medications and potential drug-drug interactions.

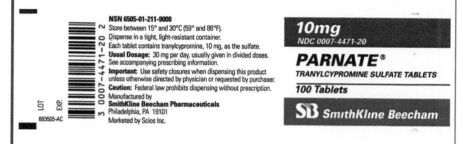

Pertinent information provided: ½ gr/d; 3 dose/d; 10 mg/tab
Unit equivalency conversion: 60 mg/gr
Desired unit: tab/dose

CORRECT setup:

$$\frac{tab}{10\ mg} \times \frac{60\ mg}{gr} \times \frac{1\ gr}{2\ d} \times \frac{d}{3\ dose} = 1\ tab/dose$$

A × U × O × Os = Ans

Selective Serotonin Reuptake Inhibitors

EXAMPLE 5

Ordered: Paxil 20 mg PO q.d.
Available: Paroxetine HCl ⅓-gr tab

Calculate the number of tab/dose.

The conversion factor for ⅓ gr/tab is:

$$\frac{1\ gr}{3\ tab}$$

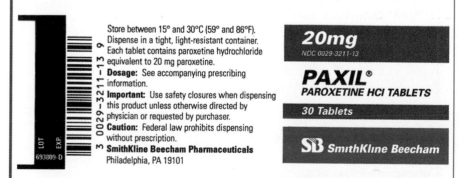

Pertinent information provided: 20 mg/dose; ⅓ gr/tab
Unit equivalency conversion: 60 mg/gr
Desired unit: tab/dose

$A \times U \times O = Ans$

Answer: Calculate the mg/dose and select the dosage form as indicated.

$O \times Os = Ans$

Venlafaxine 75-mg tab meets the order with 1 tab/dose.

If a tab is not scored, it may break unevenly, resulting in an inaccurate dose and waste.

Assess the potential side and adverse effects of the medication administered. Provide information to the patient, family members, and caregivers about possible side and adverse effects of medications.

$A \times O = Ans$

Be sure to note that 200 mg/d (per day) is ordered for your patient and given b.i.d. This is different from 200 mg b.i.d.

CORRECT setup:

$$\frac{3 \text{ tab}}{1 \text{ gr}} \times \frac{\text{gr}}{60 \text{ mg}} \times \frac{20 \text{ mg}}{\text{dose}} = 1 \text{ tab/dose}$$

E X A M P L E   6

Ordered: Effexor 225 mg/d PO t.i.d.
Available: Venlafaxine in dosage forms of 37.5 mg, 75 mg, and 100 mg
Which one of the available dosage forms will be most suitable?

M I N I   Q U I Z
What is this problem asking you to do?

Pertinent information provided: 225 mg/d; 3 dose/d
Unit equivalency conversion: None needed
Desired unit: mg/dose

CORRECT setup:

$$\frac{225 \text{ mg}}{\text{d}} \times \frac{\text{d}}{3 \text{ dose}} = 75 \text{ mg/dose}$$

Answer: The most appropriate dosage form will be the venlafaxine 75-mg tab. Venlafaxine 37.5 mg will require 2 tab/dose. Venlafaxine 100 mg will necessitate cutting the tab into an awkward dose size of ¾ tab. It is difficult to divide tab into quarters accurately.

Tetracyclic Agents

E X A M P L E   7

Ordered: Ludiomil 75 mg q.h.s.
Available: Maprotiline HCl 50-mg tab

Calculate the number of tab/dose.
Pertinent information provided: 75 mg/dose; 50 mg/tab
Unit equivalency conversion: None needed
Desired unit: tab/dose

CORRECT setup:

$$\frac{\text{tab}}{50 \text{ mg}} \times \frac{75 \text{ mg}}{\text{dose}} = 1\frac{1}{2} \text{ tab/dose}$$

Derivatives of Other Chemical Classes

E X A M P L E   8

Ordered: Wellbutrin 200 mg/d PO b.i.d.
Available: Bupropion HCl 100-mg tab

Calculate the number of tab/dose.

Pertinent information provided: 200 mg/d; 2 dose/d; 100 mg/tab
Unit equivalency conversion: None needed
Desired unit: tab/dose

CORRECT setup:

$$\frac{\text{tab}}{100 \text{ mg}} \times \frac{200 \text{ mg}}{\text{d}} \times \frac{\text{d}}{2 \text{ dose}} = 1 \text{ tab/dose}$$

 A × Ord × Os = Ans

EXAMPLE 9

Ordered: Desyrel 150 mg PO q.d.
Available: Trazodone HCl 5-gr tab

Calculate the number of tab/dose.
Pertinent information provided: 150 mg/dose; 5 gr/tab
Unit equivalency conversion: 60 mg/gr
Desired unit: tab/dose

CORRECT setup:

$$\frac{\text{tab}}{5 \text{ gr}} \times \frac{\text{gr}}{60 \text{ mg}} \times \frac{150 \text{ mg}}{\text{dose}} = \frac{1}{2} \text{ tab/dose}$$

 A × U × O = Ans

CALCULATIONS FOR ADMINISTRATION OF LITHIUM AND MOOD-NORMALIZING MEDICATIONS

The following are examples of dosage calculations for the administration of lithium and mood-normalizing agents.

EXAMPLE 1

Ordered: Eskalith 300 mg PO t.i.d.
Available: Lithium carbonate 300-mg capsules (cap)

Calculate the number of cap/dose.
Pertinent information provided: 300 mg/dose; 300 mg/cap
Unit equivalency conversion: None needed
Desired unit: cap/dose

 Instruct patients on the importance of medication compliance in achieving and maintaining therapeutic dosages.

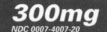

NSN 6505-00-482-8058
Store between 15° and 30°C (59° and 86°F).
Dispense in a tight container. Each capsule
contains lithium carbonate, 300 mg.
Usual Dosage: 1 or 2 capsules t.i.d.
See accompanying prescribing information.
Important: Use safety closures when
dispensing this product unless otherwise
directed by physician or requested by
purchaser.
Caution: Federal law prohibits dispensing
without prescription.
Manufactured by
SmithKline Beecham Pharmaceuticals
Philadelphia, PA 19101
Marketed by Scios Inc.

LOT
EXP.
693497-T

3 0007-4007-20 3

300mg
NDC 0007-4007-20

ESKALITH®

**LITHIUM CARBONATE
CAPSULES**

100 Capsules

SB SmithKline Beecham

$A \times O = \text{Ans}$

$\text{Ord} = 300 \text{ mg/d}$
$\text{Os} = 3 \text{ dose/d}$

CORRECT setup:

$$\frac{\text{cap}}{300 \text{ mg}} \times \frac{300 \text{ mg}}{3 \text{ dose}} = 1 \text{ cap/dose}$$

E X A M P L E   2

Ordered: Lithium citrate 300 mg/d PO t.i.d.
Available: Lithium citrate 300 mg/5 ml

Calculate the number of ml/dose.

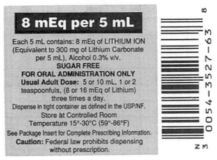

NDC 0054-3527-63   500 mL

LITHIUM
Citrate
Syrup USP

8 mEq per 5 mL

Each 5 mL contains: 8 mEq of LITHIUM ION
(Equivalent to 300 mg of Lithium Carbonate
per 5 mL), Alcohol 0.3% v/v.
SUGAR FREE
FOR ORAL ADMINISTRATION ONLY
Usual Adult Dose: 5 or 10 mL, 1 or 2
teaspoonfuls, (8 or 16 mEq of Lithium)
three times a day.
Dispense in tight container as defined in the USP/NF.
Store at Controlled Room
Temperature 15°-30°C (59°-86°F)
See Package Insert for Complete Prescribing Information.
Caution: Federal law prohibits dispensing
without prescription.

LITHIUM CITRATE SYRUP USP, 8 mEq per 5 mL
Store at Controlled Room Temperature 15°-30°C (59°-86°F)

LOT
EXP.

NSN 6505-01-168-0537   Roxane Laboratories, Inc. Columbus, Ohio 43216   4121000 033 © RLI, 1993

Pertinent information provided: 300 mg/d; 3 dose/d; 300 mg/5 ml
Unit equivalency conversion: None needed
Desired unit: ml/dose

CORRECT setup:

$A \times \text{Ord} \times \text{Os} = \text{Ans}$

$$\frac{5 \text{ ml}}{300 \text{ mg}} \times \frac{300 \text{ mg}}{\text{d}} \times \frac{\text{d}}{3 \text{ dose}} = 1.66 = 1.7 \text{ ml/dose}$$

E X A M P L E   3

Ordered: Depakene 250 mg PO t.i.d.
Available: Valproic acid syrup 250 mg/5 ml

Calculate the number of tsp/d.
Pertinent information provided: 250 mg/dose; 3 dose/d; 250 mg/5 ml
Unit equivalency conversion: 5 ml/tsp
Desired unit: tsp/d

CORRECT setup:

$U \times A \times O \times \text{Os} = \text{Ans}$

$$\frac{\text{tsp}}{5 \text{ ml}} \times \frac{5 \text{ ml}}{250 \text{ mg}} \times \frac{250 \text{ mg}}{\text{dose}} \times \frac{3 \text{ dose}}{\text{d}} = 3 \text{ tsp/d}$$

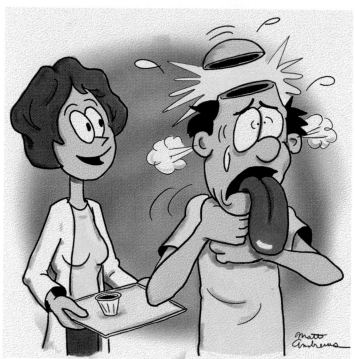

"I THINK THEY MADE THIS MEDICATION TASTE BETTER
THAN IT USED TO, DON'T YOU, MR. WRIGHT?"

EXAMPLE 4

Ordered: Tegretol 400 mg/d PO b.i.d.
Available: Carbamazepine 100-mg chewable tab

Calculate the number of tab/d.
Pertinent information provided: 400 mg/d; 100 mg/tab
Unit equivalency conversion: None needed
Desired unit: tab/d

CORRECT setup:

$$\frac{tab}{100 \text{ mg}} \times \frac{400 \text{ mg}}{d} = 4 \text{ tab/d}$$

 Be sure to read the problem carefully, noting that 400 mg/d of Tegretol is ordered, to be given in a b.i.d. dose.

 A × O = Ans

CALCULATIONS FOR ADMINISTRATION OF ANXIOLYTIC MEDICATIONS

The following are examples of dosage calculations for administration of anti-anxiety medications.

 Don't be lulled into expecting patients to behave rationally. Safety is the first rule in psychiatric nursing. Keep the patient safe. Keep others safe. Keep yourself safe.

EXAMPLE 1

Ordered: Librium 25 mg IM q.i.d.
Available: Chlordiazepoxide HCl in a 100 mg/ml ampule

Calculate the number of ml/dose.

Pertinent information provided: 25 mg/dose; 100 mg/ml
Unit equivalency conversion: None needed
Desired unit: ml/dose

CORRECT setup:

$$\frac{ml}{100 \; \cancel{mg}} \times \frac{25 \; \cancel{mg}}{dose} = 0.25 \; ml/dose$$

A × O = Ans

E X A M P L E　2

Ordered: Valium 5 mg IM q4hr p.r.n.
Available: Diazepam 5 mg/ml

Calculate the number of ml/dose.
　Pertinent information provided: 5 mg/dose; 5 mg/ml
　Unit equivalency conversion: None needed
　Desired unit: ml/dose

Take the time to study each medication. Find out how long it takes to achieve therapeutic effects and how long the effects are expected to last.

CORRECT setup:

$$\frac{ml}{5 \; \cancel{mg}} \times \frac{5 \; \cancel{mg}}{dose} = 1 \; ml/dose$$

A × O = Ans

E X A M P L E　3

Ordered: Ativan 10 mg/d IM q.i.d.
Available: Lorazepam in vials of 40 mg/10 ml

Calculate the number of ml/dose.
　Pertinent information provided: 10 mg/d; 4 dose/d; 40 mg/10 ml
　Unit equivalency conversion: None needed
　Desired unit: ml/dose

Round the calculated values to the nearest measurable unit.

CORRECT setup:

$$\frac{10 \; ml}{40 \; \cancel{mg}} \times \frac{10 \; \cancel{mg}}{\cancel{d}} \times \frac{\cancel{d}}{4 \; dose} = 0.625 = 0.63 \; ml/dose$$

A × Ord × Os = Ans

E X A M P L E　4

Ordered: Xanax 0.75 mg/d PO t.i.d.
Available: Alprazolam 250-μg tab

Calculate the number of tab/dose.

NSN 6505-01-197-3966
See Package Insert for
Complete Prescribing Information

Store at Controlled Room
Temperature 15°-30°C (59°-86°F)

PROTECT FROM MOISTURE

Dispense in a tight,
light-resistant container
as defined in the USP/NF.
Keep container tightly closed.

TABLETS IDENTIFIED

54 512

NDC 0054-
4104-29　　500 Tablets

0.25 mg (IV)

ALPRAZOLAM
Tablets USP

Each tablet contains
Alprazolam USP 0.25 mg

Caution: Federal law prohibits
dispensing without prescription.

Roxane
Laboratories, Inc.
Columbus, Ohio 43216

LOT
EXP.

4142600
043
© RLI, 1993

Pertinent information provided: 0.75 mg/d; 3 dose/d; 250 μg/tab
Unit equivalency conversion: 1000 μg/mg
Desired unit: tab/dose

CORRECT setup:

$$\frac{tab}{250\ \cancel{\mu g}} \times \frac{1000\ \cancel{\mu g}}{\cancel{mg}} \times \frac{0.75\ \cancel{mg}}{\cancel{d}} \times \frac{\cancel{d}}{3\ dose} = 1\ tab/dose$$

 A × U × Ord × Os = Ans

E X A M P L E   5

Ordered: BuSpar 30 mg/d PO b.i.d.
Available: Buspirone 15-mg tab

Calculate the number of tab/dose.

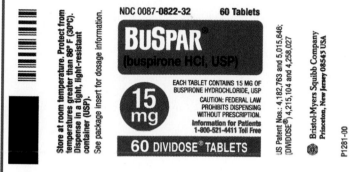

Pertinent information provided: 30 mg/d; 2 dose/d; 15 mg/tab
Unit equivalency conversion: None needed
Desired unit: tab/dose

CORRECT setup:

$$\frac{tab}{15\ \cancel{mg}} \times \frac{30\ \cancel{mg}}{\cancel{d}} \times \frac{\cancel{d}}{2\ dose} = 1\ tab/dose$$

 A × Ord × Os = Ans

CALCULATIONS FOR ADMINISTRATION OF ANTIPSYCHOTIC MEDICATIONS

Antipsychotic medications are ordered with dosages adjusted to meet the individual patient's needs, depending on the chronicity and the severity of the mental condition. The following examples illustrate dosage calculations for administration of antipsychotic drugs. The dosages presented are those recommended for the initial dosing of the respective antipsychotic medications.

 A medication dosage in a concentrated form added to fruit juice is an effective method of administration for patients who will not accept oral medications in pill form.

The Phenothiazines

E X A M P L E   1

Ordered: Thorazine ¼ mg/lb PO q.i.d. p.r.n. for severe behavioral problems
Available: Chlorpromazine 10 mg/5 ml

Your patient weighs 86 lb.
Calculate the number of ml/dose.

 The reference dose for Thorazine is in mg/lb.

An intramuscular injection of Thorazine must be given slowly, deep into the upper outer quadrant at the gluteal site.

Ord = ¼ mg/lb

NSN 6505-01-156-1640
Store below 25°C (77°F). Dispense in a tight, light-resistant glass bottle. Each 5 mL (1 teaspoon) contains chlorpromazine hydrochloride, 10 mg.
Usual Dosage: Children: 10 to 60 mg daily. Adults: 20 to 150 mg daily. See accompanying prescribing information.
Important: Use child-resistant closures when dispensing this product unless otherwise directed by physician or requested by purchaser.
Caution: Federal law prohibits dispensing without prescription.
Manufactured by
SmithKline Beecham Pharmaceuticals
Philadelphia, PA 19101
Marketed by Scios Inc.

LOT   EXP.
692563-AF

10mg/5mL
NDC 0007-5072-44

THORAZINE®
CHLORPROMAZINE
HCl SYRUP

4 fl oz (118 mL)

SB SmithKline Beecham

Pertinent information provided: ¼ mg/lb; 86 lb; 10 mg/5 ml
Unit equivalency conversion: None needed
Desired unit: ml/dose

CORRECT setup:

$$\frac{5 \text{ ml}}{10 \text{ mg}} \times \frac{1 \text{ mg}}{4 \text{ lb}} \times 86 \text{ lb} = 10.75 = 10.8 \text{ ml/dose}$$

A × Ord × BW = Ans

E X A M P L E   2

Ordered: Prolixin 1.25 mg IM t.i.d.
Available: Fluphenazine HCl 2.5 mg/ml

10 mL MULTIPLE DOSE   NDC 0003-0586-30
2.5 mg per mL
PROLIXIN® INJECTION
Fluphenazine Hydrochloride Injection USP
Sterile • Intramuscular
See insert for dosage information
Caution: Federal law prohibits dispensing without prescription
Protect from light
Store at room temperature; avoid freezing
APOTHECON®
A Bristol-Myers Squibb Company
Princeton, NJ 08540 USA

Beware of drug-drug interactions with polypharmaceutical dosage regimens.

A × O = Ans

Calculate the number of ml/dose.
Pertinent information provided: 1.25 mg/dose; 2.5 mg/ml
Unit equivalency conversion: None needed
Desired unit: ml/dose

CORRECT setup:

$$\frac{\text{ml}}{2.5 \text{ mg}} \times \frac{1.25 \text{ mg}}{\text{dose}} = \frac{1}{2} \text{ ml/dose}$$

E X A M P L E   3

Ordered: Mellaril 50 mg PO t.i.d.
Available: Thioridazine HCl 30 mg/ml

Calculate the number of ml/dose.
Pertinent information provided: 50 mg/dose; 30 mg/ml
Unit equivalency conversion: None needed
Desired unit: ml/dose

CORRECT setup:

$$\frac{\text{ml}}{30 \text{ mg}} \times \frac{50 \text{ mg}}{\text{dose}} = 1.66 = 1.7 \text{ ml/dose}$$

 A × O = Ans

Butyrophenone

> ### E X A M P L E   4
>
> **Ordered:** Haldol 50 mg IM q.d.
> **Available:** Haloperidol decanoate 500 mg/5 ml
>
> Calculate the number of ml/dose.
>   **Pertinent information provided:** 50 mg/dose; 500 mg/5 ml
>   **Unit equivalency conversion:** None needed
>   **Desired unit:** ml/dose
>
> *CORRECT* setup:
>
> $$\frac{5 \text{ ml}}{500 \text{ mg}} \times \frac{50 \text{ mg}}{\text{dose}} = \frac{1}{2} \text{ ml/dose}$$

 Inject Haldol with a 21-G 1½ in. (or longer) needle for deep intramuscular administration.

 A × O = Ans

Thioxanthene

> ### E X A M P L E   5
>
> **Ordered:** Navane 1 ml PO b.i.d.
> **Available:** Thiothixene HCl concentrate with an accompanying dropper calibrated at 2, 3, 4, 5, 6, 8, and 10 mg (5 mg/ml)
>
> Calculate the number of mg/dose.
>   **Pertinent information provided:** 1 ml/dose; 5 mg/ml
>   **Unit equivalency conversion:** None needed
>   **Desired unit:** mg/dose
>
> *CORRECT* setup:
>
> $$\frac{5 \text{ mg}}{\text{ml}} \times \frac{1 \text{ ml}}{\text{dose}} = 5 \text{ mg/dose}$$

 Medication droppers are frequently lost or destroyed, so you will need to use available volume measures (that is, syringes) to continue the administration of the remaining dosages.

 A × O = Ans

Oxoindole

> ### E X A M P L E   6
>
> **Ordered:** Moban 60 mg/d PO t.i.d.
> **Available:** Molindone HCl 10-mg tab
>
> Calculate the number of tab/dose.
>   **Pertinent information provided:** 60 mg/d 3 dose/d; 10 mg/tab
>   **Unit equivalency conversion:** None needed
>   **Desired unit:** tab/dose
>
> *CORRECT* setup:
>
> $$\frac{\text{tab}}{10 \text{ mg}} \times \frac{60 \text{ mg}}{\text{d}} \times \frac{\text{d}}{3 \text{ dose}} = 2 \text{ tab/dose}$$

 A × Ord × Os = Ans

Dibenzoxazepine

Mix oral concentrates
with orange or grapefruit
juice prior to administration, to disguise their un-
palatable taste and pro-
vide a medium for
enhancing absorption.

A × O = Ans

E X A M P L E   7

Ordered: Loxitane 10 mg PO b.i.d.
Available: Loxapine HCl oral concentrate 25 mg/ml

Calculate the number of ml/dose.
   Pertinent information provided: 10 mg/dose; 25 mg/ml
   Unit equivalency conversion: None needed
   Desired unit: ml/dose

CORRECT setup:

$$\frac{\text{ml}}{25 \ \text{mg}} \times \frac{10 \ \text{mg}}{\text{dose}} = 0.4 \ \text{ml/dose}$$

Dibenzodiazepine

E X A M P L E   8

Ordered: Serentil 25 mg IM now and repeat in 30 min p.r.n.
Available: Mesoridazine besylate in ampules of 25 mg/ml

Calculate the number of ml/dose.
   Pertinent information provided: 25 mg/dose; 25 mg/ml
   Unit equivalency conversion: None needed
   Desired unit: ml/dose

CORRECT setup:

$$\frac{\text{ml}}{25 \ \text{mg}} \times \frac{25 \ \text{mg}}{\text{dose}} = 1 \ \text{ml/dose}$$

A × O = Ans

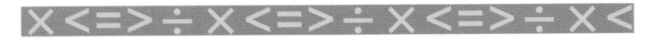

Chapter Summary

The examples in this chapter represent psychotropic agents commonly ordered for the treatment of psychiatric disorders. These dosages were arranged in categories according to their therapeutic functions. In reality, chemotherapeutic treatments of psychiatric disorders usually involve one or more classes of medications used concurrently. Moreover, patients with underlying acute or chronic conditions may require additional medication dosages for situations such as infection control, hypertension, or bronchial asthma.

If you cannot follow the examples presented in this chapter, you should review Chapters 4 and 5, because most medications used in psychiatry are ordered as oral and/or injection dosages. Again, you are reminded to research all medications you are not familiar with before administering them to your patients. You will also need to carry out pertinent nursing interventions for each dosage administered. Information on side effects and adverse reactions to medications was not provided because it falls within the domain of pharmacology.

PROBLEM SET	PROBLEM SET ANSWERS
1. Ordered: Moban 10 mg PO t.i.d. Available: Molindone HCl 20 mg/ml Calculate the number of ml/dose.	1. 0.5 ml/dose
2. Ordered: Versed 5 mg IVSP q 2hr p.r.n. Available: Midazolam HCl 5 mg/ml Calculate the number of ml/dose.	2. 1 ml/dose
3. Ordered: Antabuse 500 mg PO q.d. Available: Disulfiram 250-mg tab Calculate the number of tab/dose.	3. 2 tab/dose
4. Ordered: Sinequan 150 mg PO q.h.s. Available: Doxepin HCl 75-mg capsule (cap) Calculate the number of cap/dose.	4. 2 cap/dose
5. Ordered: Mellaril 50 mg PO t.i.d. Available: Thioridazine HCl 100 mg/ml suspension Calculate the number of ml/dose.	5. 0.5 ml/dose

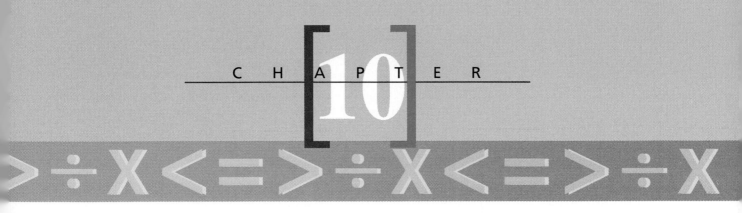

Elderly Population: Medication Calculation Using Dimensional Analysis

INTRODUCTION

In this chapter, dosage calculations for the administration of medications to the elderly population will be discussed. The process of dosage calculation with dimensional analysis (DA) follows the examples presented in Unit I, but the examples in this chapter represent medications commonly ordered for the elderly population. The emphasis is on specific types of illnesses and the individual elderly patient's needs.

Again, you are reminded that applying DA to dosage calculations frees you from having to remember any formulas, regardless of drug, dosage form, or route of administration. When you use DA your focus will remain on extracting the pertinent information from the problem and setting up the conversion factors that enable you to cancel unwanted units. Of course, accuracy in math is an absolute essential when you are calculating medication dosages.

LEARNING OBJECTIVES

By the end of this chapter, you will be able to calculate medication dosages using DA for the administration of medications in:

- Cardiac care

- Pulmonary conditions

- Chronic neurologic conditions

- Chronic joint disorders and pain control

CALCULATIONS FOR DRUG ADMINISTRATION IN CARDIAC CARE

The following examples demonstrate DA in the calculation of medications that are frequently ordered for patients who need cardiac care.

Nitroglycerin orders are frequently given in grains (gr).

Read the order carefully, and do not confuse gr with gm.

E X A M P L E   1

Your patient has angina.

> **Ordered:** Nitroglycerin ¹⁄₁₅₀ gr SL q5min until pain free, p.r.n., up to 3 tab
> **Available:** Nitrostat* SL 0.4-mg tab

Calculate the number of tab/dose.

Patient Information Enclosed

N 0071-0570-13

Nitrostat®
(Nitroglycerin Tablets, USP)
0.4 mg (1/150 gr)

Caution—Federal law prohibits dispensing without prescription.

4 PACK

100 Sublingual Tablets
(4 bottles of 25 tablets each)

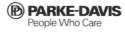

Ⓟ **PARKE-DAVIS**
People Who Care

Nitrostat® (Nitroglycerin Tablets, USP)   0.4 mg (1/150 gr)

*Nitrostat® is a registered trademark of Warner-Lambert Company.

Pertinent information provided: $\frac{1}{150}$ gr/dose; 0.4 mg/tab
Unit equivalency conversion: 60 mg/gr
Desired unit: tab/dose

CORRECT setup:

$$\frac{\text{tab}}{0.4 \text{ mg}} \times \frac{60 \text{ mg}}{\text{gr}} \times \frac{1 \text{ gr}}{150 \text{ dose}} = 1 \text{ tab/dose}$$

 A × U × O = Ans

E X A M P L E   2

Your patient is undergoing thrombolytic therapy.
    Ordered: Aspirin 5 gr chew and swallow stat and q.d.
    Available: Aspirin 81-mg chewable tab

Calculate the number of tab/dose.
    Pertinent information provided: 5 gr/dose; 81 mg/tab
    Unit equivalency conversion: 60 to 65 mg/gr
    Desired unit: tab/dose

 Aspirin, Tylenol, and FeSO$_4$ are other examples of medication ordered in gr.

 Be sensitive to bitter- or sour-tasting medication. Give the patient some apple juice or sherbet to cleanse the palate.

CORRECT setup:

$$\frac{\text{tab}}{81 \text{ mg}} \times \frac{60 \text{ to } 65 \text{ mg}}{\text{gr}} \times \frac{5 \text{ gr}}{\text{dose}} = 3.70 \text{ to } 4.01 = 4 \text{ tab/dose}$$

 A × U × O = Ans

E X A M P L E   3

Your patient has hypertension.
    Ordered: Norvasc 5 mg PO q.d.
    Available: Amlodipine 10-mg tab

Calculate the number of tab/dose.
    Pertinent information provided: 5 mg/dose; 10 mg/tab
    Unit equivalency conversion: None needed
    Desired unit: tab/dose

 A standard oral dosage order can be solved by multiplying the conversion factors of the available dosages and the ordered dosages, that is, A × O = Ans.

CORRECT setup:

$$\frac{\text{tab}}{10 \text{ mg}} \times \frac{5 \text{ mg}}{\text{dose}} = \frac{1}{2} \text{ tab/dose}$$

E X A M P L E   4

Your patient has congestive heart failure.
    Ordered: Bumex 1 mg IVSP q2hr (max 10 mg/d)
    Available: Bumetanide in vials of 0.25 mg/ml

Calculate the number of ml/dose.
    Pertinent information provided: 1 mg/dose; 0.25 mg/ml
    Unit equivalency conversion: None needed
    Desired unit: ml/dose

 Round a medication dosage to the nearest measurable unit; for example, if you cannot measure 2.435 ml, then why calculate your answer to the third decimal place?

CORRECT setup:

$$\frac{\text{ml}}{0.25 \text{ mg}} \times \frac{1 \text{ mg}}{\text{dose}} = 4 \text{ ml/dose}$$

 A × O = Ans

DF = 15 gtt/ml
Or = 1 L/hr for NS
   = 150 ml/hr
      for D$_5$ ½ NS

DF × U × Or × U =
Ans

DF × Or × U = Ans

DF = 15 gtt/ml
Or = 70 mg/hr
A = 500 mg
Av = 100, 250, or
500 ml

DF × A × Or × U =
Ans

18 gtt/min = 3 drop/10
sec
9 gtt/min = 3 drop/20
sec
4 gtt/min = 1 drop/15
sec

Ov = 50 ml
Ot = 30 min
DF = 15 gtt/ml
Ord = 2 mg/kg loading
dose

EXAMPLE 4

Your patient was stung by a wasp, went into anaphylactic shock, and was brought to the urgent care unit.

Ordered: Epinephrine 1% (10 mg/ml) 0.3 ml SQ q10min with LR 1 L/hr, followed by D$_5$ ½ NS at 150 ml/hr

Calculate the drip rate of LR and D$_5$ ½ NS in gtt/min (15 gtt/ml).
Pertinent information provided: 1 L/hr; 150 ml/hr; 15 gtt/ml
Unit equivalency conversion: 1000 ml/L
Desired unit: gtt/min

CORRECT setup:

1. NS:

$$\frac{15\ gtt}{ml} \times \frac{1000\ ml}{L} \times \frac{1\ L}{hr} \times \frac{hr}{60\ min} = 250\ gtt/min$$

2. D$_5$ ½ NS:

$$\frac{15\ gtt}{ml} \times \frac{150\ ml}{hr} \times \frac{hr}{60\ min} = 35.5 = 36\ gtt/min$$

EXAMPLE 5

Your patient has had a severe allergic response.

Ordered: Hydrocortisone sodium succinate 500 mg at 70 mg/hr continuous IV infusion

Available: Solu-Cortef in vials of 500 mg/ml, with a macrodrop administration system (15 gtt/ml), and D$_5$W in 100-ml, 250-ml, and 500-ml bags

Calculate which of the D$_5$W dosage forms will be appropriate for this order.
Pertinent information provided: 500 mg/dose; 70 mg/hr; 15 gtt/ml
Unit equivalency conversion: None needed
Desired dimension: gtt/min in 100-, 250-, and 500-ml bags

CORRECT setup:

$$\frac{15\ gtt}{ml} \times \frac{500\ ml}{500\ mg} \times \frac{70\ mg}{hr} \times \frac{hr}{60\ min} = 17.5 = 18\ gtt/min$$

$$\frac{15\ gtt}{ml} \times \frac{250\ ml}{500\ mg} \times \frac{70\ mg}{hr} \times \frac{hr}{60\ min} = 8.75 = 9\ gtt/min$$

$$\frac{15\ gtt}{ml} \times \frac{100\ ml}{500\ mg} \times \frac{70\ mg}{hr} \times \frac{hr}{60\ min} = 3.5 = 4\ gtt/min$$

Answer: Either the 250- or 500-ml bag can be used in this order.

EXAMPLE 6

Your patient, who weighs 224 lb, has pneumonia.

Ordered: Tobramycin loading dose of 2 mg/kg in D$_5$W 50 ml IVPB over 30 min (15 gtt/ml) plus a maintenance dose of tobramycin 1.7 mg/kg in D$_5$W 50 ml IV q8hr

Available: Tobramycin in vials of 80 mg/2 ml

1. Calculate the number of mg/dose for a loading dose of 2 mg/kg.
2a. Calculate the flow rate in ml/hr.
 b. Calculate the number of gtt/min.
3. Calculate the number of mg/dose at 1.7 mg/kg.

Pertinent information provided: 2 mg/kg; 50 ml/dose; 30 min/dose; 224 lb; 1.7 mg/kg

Unit equivalency conversion: 2.2 lb/kg

Desired units: (1) mg/dose loading dose (2 mg/kg); (2a) ml/hr; (2b) gtt/min; (3) mg/dose of maintenance at 1.7 mg/kg

CORRECT setup:

1. mg/dose (loading dose):

$$\frac{2\text{ mg}}{\text{kg}} \times \frac{\text{kg}}{2.2\text{ lb}} \times 224\text{ lb} = 203.64 = 204\text{ mg}$$

 Ord × U × BW = Ans

2a. ml/hr

$$\frac{50\text{ ml}}{\text{dose}} \times \frac{\text{dose}}{30\text{ min}} \times \frac{60\text{ min}}{\text{hr}} = 100\text{ ml/hr}$$

 Ov × Ot × U = Ans

 b. gtt/min:

$$\frac{15\text{ gtt}}{\text{ml}} \times \frac{50\text{ ml}}{\text{dose}} \times \frac{\text{dose}}{30\text{ min}} = 25\text{ gtt/min}$$

 DF × Ov × Ot = Ans

3. mg/dose:

$$\frac{1.7\text{ mg}}{\text{kg}} \times \frac{\text{kg}}{2.2\text{ lb}} \times 224\text{ lb} = 173.09 = 173\text{ mg/dose}$$

 Ord × U × BW = Ans

Available is tobramycin 1.2 gm/30 ml.

1. Calculate the number of ml/dose for the loading dose (2 mg/kg).
2. Calculate the number of ml/dose for the maintenance dose (1.7 mg/kg).

1. Loading dose:

$$\frac{204\text{ mg}}{\text{dose}} \times \frac{\text{gm}}{1000\text{ mg}} \times \frac{30\text{ ml}}{1.2\text{ gm}} = 5.1\text{ ml/dose}$$

 O × U × A = Ans

2. Maintenance:

$$\frac{30\text{ ml}}{1.2\text{ gm}} \times \frac{\text{gm}}{1000\text{ mg}} \times \frac{173\text{ mg}}{\text{dose}} = 4.3\text{ ml/dose}$$

 A × U × O = Ans

CALCULATIONS FOR DRUG ADMINISTRATION IN CHRONIC NEUROLOGIC CONDITIONS

The following are examples of medication dosage calculations for administration in chronic neurologic disorders.

Do not cut or crush tab-
lets, caplets, or capsules
that are designed to re-
lease medication over a
period of time, for exam-
ple, ER, SR, XL.

A × O = Ans

In the first 3 days, the
patient will receive the
larger dose, then, for the
balance of the month (or
the next 27 days), the patient will receive the
smaller dose.

A × Ord × Ot + A ×
Ord × Ot = Ans

PR = rectal administra-
tion (per rectum)

A × O = Ans

Dilute ml/dose of Depa-
kene with 1 part of water
for the total volume.

E X A M P L E   1

Ordered: Ticlid 250 mg PO b.i.d.
Available: Ticlopidine HCl 250-mg tab

Calculate the number of tab/dose.
  Pertinent information provided: 250 mg/tab; 250 mg/dose
  Unit equivalency conversion: None needed
  Desired unit: tab/dose

CORRECT setup:

$$\frac{tab}{250 \ mg} \times \frac{250 \ mg}{dose} = 1 \ tab/dose$$

E X A M P L E   2

Ordered: Coumadin loading dose of 5 mg PO q.d. for 3 d, and then
        maintainenance dose of Coumadin 2 mg PO q.d.
Available: Warfarin sodium 2-mg tab

Calculate the number of tab for 30 d of treatment.
  Pertinent information provided: 5 mg/d; 3 d; 2 mg/d; balance of 30 d; 2
    mg/tab
  Unit equivalency conversion: None needed
  Desired unit: tab/30 d of treatment

CORRECT setup:

$$\left[\frac{tab}{2 \ mg} \times \frac{5 \ mg}{d} \times 3 \ d\right] + \left[\frac{tab}{2 \ mg} \times \frac{2 \ mg}{d} \times 27 \ d\right]$$
$$= 7\tfrac{1}{2} \ tab + 27 \ tab = 34\tfrac{1}{2} = 35 \ tab$$

E X A M P L E   3

Ordered: Valproate 200 mg diluted 1 : 1 in tap water per rectum (PR) as a
        retention enema
Available: Depakene 250 mg/5 ml

1. Calculate the number of ml of Depakene/dose.
2. Calculate the total number of ml/dose.

  Pertinent information provided: 200 mg/dose; 250 mg/5 ml
  Unit equivalency conversion: None needed
  Desired units: ml/dose Depakene; total ml/dose

CORRECT setup:

1. ml/dose:

$$\frac{5 \ ml}{250 \ mg} \times \frac{200 \ mg}{dose} = 4 \ ml/dose$$

2. total ml/dose:

   1 : 1 dilution = 4 ml Depakene in 4 ml tap water = 8 ml/dose total volume

EXAMPLE 4

Your patient has increased intracranial pressure.
   Ordered: Mannitol 100 mg IV bolus over 20 min
   Available: Mannitol 100 mg in D$_5$W 50 ml

Calculate the flow rate in ml/hr.
   Pertinent information provided: 100 mg/dose; 20 min/dose; 100 mg/50 ml
   Unit equivalency conversion: 60 min/hr
   Desired unit: ml/hr

CORRECT setup:

$$\frac{50 \text{ ml}}{100 \text{ mg}} \times \frac{100 \text{ mg}}{\text{dose}} \times \frac{\text{dose}}{20 \text{ min}} \times \frac{60 \text{ min}}{\text{hr}} = 150 \text{ ml/hr}$$

Mannitol is frequently infused at a rapid rate.

A × O × Ot × U = Ans

EXAMPLE 5

Your patient, who weighs 153 lb, suffers from epilepsy.
   Ordered: Phenytoin 10 mg/kg loading dose IVSP at 30 mg/min
   Available: Dilantin in vials of 250 mg/5 ml

1. Calculate the number of ml of Dilantin/dose in the loading dose.
2. Calculate the number of min to administer the order.

   Pertinent information provided: 10 mg/kg; 153 lb; 250 mg/5 ml; 30 mg/min
   Unit equivalency conversion: 2.2 lb/kg
   Desired units: (1) ml of Dilantin/loading dose (2) IVSP min/dose

CORRECT setup:

1. ml of Dilantin/loading dose:

$$\frac{5 \text{ ml}}{250 \text{ mg}} \times \frac{10 \text{ mg}}{\text{kg}} \times \frac{\text{kg}}{2.2 \text{ lb}} \times 153 \text{ lb} = 13.9 = 14 \text{ ml}$$

2. number of min to administer the order:

$$\frac{\text{min}}{30 \text{ mg}} \times \frac{250 \text{ mg}}{5 \text{ ml}} \times \frac{14 \text{ ml}}{\text{dose}} = 23 \text{ min/dose}$$

It would be easier to administer this order IVPB.

Dilantin (phenytoin) *cannot* be mixed in a solution containing glucose or dextrose (D$_5$W).

Ord = 10 mg/kg
Or = 30 mg/min
A = 250 mg/5 ml

A × Ord × U × BW = Ans

Or × A × Ov = Ans

CALCULATIONS FOR ADMINISTRATION IN CHRONIC JOINT DISORDERS AND IN PAIN CONTROL

The following are examples of medication dosage calculations for administration in chronic joint disorders and pain control.

E X A M P L E   1

Ordered: Toradol 60 mg IM stat
Available: Ketorolac tromethamine in 30 mg/ml Tubex single-dose cartridges

Calculate the number of ml/dose.
Pertinent information provided: 60 mg/dose; 30 mg/ml
Unit equivalency conversion: None needed
Desired unit: ml/dose

CORRECT setup:

 A × O = Ans

$$\frac{ml}{30 \text{ mg}} \times \frac{60 \text{ mg}}{dose} = 2 \text{ ml/dose}$$

E X A M P L E   2

Ordered: Naprosyn 500 mg PO b.i.d.
Available: Naproxen 250-mg tab

Calculate the number of tab/d.

Os = t.i.d. = 3 dose/d

NSN 6505-01-026-9730
Usual Dosage: See Package Insert
for Complete Prescribing Information

Store at Controlled Room
Temperature 15°-30°C (59°-86°F)

PROTECT FROM MOISTURE

Dispense in a well-closed,
light-resistant container
as defined in the USP/NF.

This Package Not For Household Use.
Dispense Prescriptions Using Child
Resistant Closures.

TABLETS IDENTIFIED

54 643

NDC 0054-4641-25   100 Tablets

250 mg

NAPROXEN

Tablets USP

Each tablet contains Naproxen 250 mg

Caution: Federal law prohibits
dispensing without prescription.

Roxane
Laboratories, Inc.
Columbus, Ohio 43216

4180710
115
© RLI, 1995

Pertinent information provided: 500 mg/dose; 250 mg/tab; 2 dose/d
Unit equivalency conversion: None needed
Desired unit: tab/d

CORRECT setup:

 A × O × Os = Ans

$$\frac{tab}{250 \text{ mg}} \times \frac{500 \text{ mg}}{dose} \times \frac{2 \text{ dose}}{d} = 4 \text{ tab/d}$$

E X A M P L E   3

Ordered: Dolophine HCl 0.1 mg/kg (max 10 mg/dose) IM q4hr p.r.n.
Available: Methadone HCl in ampules of 10 mg/ml

Calculate the number of ml/dose for your patient, who weighs 289 lb.
Pertinent information provided: 0.1 mg/kg per dose; 10 mg/ml; 289 lb;
max 10 mg/dose
Unit equivalency conversion: 2.2 lb/kg
Desired unit: ml/dose

A dosage cannot exceed
the maximum reference
dose.

Ord = 0.1 mg/kg per
dose
Maximum reference
dose = 10 mg/dose

CORRECT setup:

$$289 \text{ lb} \times \frac{\text{kg}}{2.2 \text{ lb}} \times \frac{0.1 \text{ mg}}{\text{kg} \cdot \text{dose}} = 13.1 \text{ mg/dose}$$

13.1 mg/dose > maximum 10 mg/dose

$$\frac{\text{ml}}{10 \text{ mg}} \times \frac{10 \text{ mg}}{\text{dose}} = 1 \text{ ml/dose}$$

 BW × U × Ord = Ans

 A × O = Ans

EXAMPLE 4

Ordered: Indocin 50 mg PO q6hr × 2 d, then 50 mg PO t.i.d. × 2 d, then 25 mg PO t.i.d. for maintenance
Available: Indomethacin 50-mg tab

Calculate the number of tab for 30 d of treatment.
   Pertinent information provided: 50 mg/dose; 4 dose/d for 2 d; 3 dose/d for 2 d; 25 mg/dose; 3 dose/d for the balance of 30 d (26 d); 50 mg/ tab
   Unit equivalency conversion: None needed
   Desired unit: tab for 30 d

CORRECT setup:

$$\frac{\text{tab}}{50 \text{ mg}} \times \frac{50 \text{ mg}}{\text{dose}} \times \frac{4 \text{ dose}}{\text{d}} \times 2 \text{ d} = 8 \text{ tab for the first 2 d}$$

$$\frac{\text{tab}}{50 \text{ mg}} \times \frac{50 \text{ mg}}{\text{dose}} \times \frac{3 \text{ dose}}{\text{d}} \times 2 \text{ d} = 6 \text{ tab for the next 2 d}$$

$$\frac{\text{tab}}{50 \text{ mg}} \times \frac{25 \text{ mg}}{\text{dose}} \times \frac{3 \text{ dose}}{\text{d}} \times 26 \text{ d} = 39 \text{ tab for the balance of the mo}$$

Total number of tab needed = 8 + 6 + 39 = 53 tabs for 30 d

 Read the problem carefully.

 Medications, such as indomethacin and prednisone, are ordered in decreasing doses.

 In most cases, the pharmacy will dispense the medication as ordered. Your provider, however, may ask you to dispense the order from samples of medication received directly from pharmaceutical companies.

 A × O × Os × Ot = Ans

 Total = 8 + 6 + 39 = 53 tabs

EXAMPLE 5

Ordered: An intra-articular injection of Decadron-LA 4 mg in lidocaine to a total volume of 5 ml via a 27-G needle
Available: Decadron-LA 8 mg/ml sterile suspension

1. Calculate the number of ml/dose Decadron-LA.
2. Calculate the amount of ml/dose lidocaine.

   Pertinent information provided: 4 mg/dose; 8 mg/ml
   Unit equivalency conversion: None needed
   Desired units: (1) ml/dose Decadron-LA; (2) ml/dose lidocaine

CORRECT setup:

1. ml/dose Decadron-LA

$$\frac{\text{ml}}{8 \text{ mg}} \times \frac{4 \text{ mg}}{\text{dose}} = \frac{1}{2} \text{ ml Decadron-LA}$$

2. ml/dose lidocaine

   5 ml − 0.5 ml = 4.5 ml lidocaine

To prepare this order:
- ✔ Draw 4.5 ml lidocaine into a 6-ml syringe.
- ✔ Pull the plunger away from the needle. Remove the needle from the syringe and discard the needle.
- ✔ Take 1-ml syringe, draw 0.5 ml Decadron-LA.
- ✔ Inject 0.5 ml Decadron-LA into 6-ml syringe containing 4.5 ml lidocaine.
- ✔ Attach a 27-G needle.
- ✔ Eliminate excess air space.

 A × O = Ans

 Total vol − Decadron-LA vol = lidocaine volume

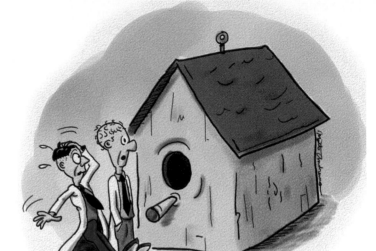

"I MUST HAVE PLACED THE DECIMAL POINT
IN THE WRONG PLACE."

Draw up the medications
as in Example 5, except
you will need to use a
30-ml syringe.

Use a 6-ml syringe to
draw 5 ml of NS for an
NS flush.

A × O = Ans

Total volume − colchi-
cine volume = NS vol-
ume

EXAMPLE 6

Ordered: Colchicine 2 mg in NS to a total of 20 ml, and 5 ml NS flush
Available: Colchicine in ampules of 1 mg/2 ml

1. Calculate the number of ml/dose colchicine.
2. Calculate the number of ml/dose NS.

Pertinent information provided: 2 mg/dose; 1 mg/2 ml
Unit equivalency conversion: None needed
Desired unit: ml/dose colchicine and NS

CORRECT setup:

1. ml/dose colchicine:

$$\frac{2 \text{ ml}}{\text{mg}} \times \frac{2 \text{ mg}}{\text{dose}} = 4 \text{ ml/dose colchicine}$$

2. ml/dose NS:

$$20 \text{ ml} - 4 \text{ ml} = 16 \text{ ml NS}$$

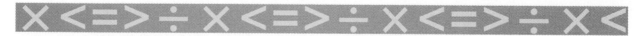

Chapter Summary

An array of dosage calculations has been presented for the administration of medications frequently ordered in the treatment of illnesses in the elderly population. The questions involve multiple steps that simulate actual orders. In institutions supported by a pharmacy, you do not have to reconstitute most IV medications, as they will be brought to you ready to administer as ordered. It is not however, guaranteed that you will have full pharmacy support at your work site. Therefore, it behooves you to be knowledgeable in calculating medication dosages for administration as ordered by the providers.

If you are having difficulty in following the examples presented in this chapter, please review the following checklist:

✔ Remember to read the problem carefully.
✔ Ask yourself if you have a clear understanding of what the problem is asking you to do.
✔ Carefully extract all pertinent information provided in the problem.
✔ Make sure the necessary unit equivalency conversion factor(s) are placed in the setup.
✔ Orient the desired dimensions properly in their numerator/denominator placements.
✔ Remember that to cancel, you must have the same units in the numerator as in the denominator.
✔ Check to make sure that the math is done accurately.

PROBLEM SET	PROBLEM SET ANSWERS
1. Ordered: Epinephrine (1 : 10,000) 0.5 mg in 10 ml NS endotracheal tube (ET) stat. Available: Epinephrine (1 : 10,000) 1 mg/ml 10-ml vial. a. Calculate the number of ml/dose. b. What is the route of administration?	1. a. ½ ml/dose b. Administer via the endotracheal tube.
2. Ordered: Acetaminophen 1 gm q.i.d. Available: Acetaminophen 325 mg/5 ml Calculate the number of tsp/dose.	2. 3 tsp/dose

PROBLEM SET	PROBLEM SET ANSWERS

3. Ordered: Solu-Medrol 125 mg IV q6hr
     Available: Methylprednisolone 40 mg/ml
     Calculate the number of ml/dose.
	3. 3.1 ml/dose

4. Ordered: Prednisone 20 mg t.i.d. for 2 d, then 20 mg b.i.d. for 2 d, then 20 mg q.d. for 2 d, then 10 mg q.o.d. for 1 wk Calculate the number of tab needed for this order.	4. 14 tab

5. Ordered: Increase the dosage of allopurinol from 300 mg PO q.d. to 400 mg PO q.d.
     Available: Allopurinol 100-mg tab
     Calculate the number of tab at the increased dose.
	5. From 3 tab now, increase to 4 tab/dose

6. Ordered: Demerol 100 mg IM q6hr p.r.n.
     Available: Meperidine HCl 50 mg/ml
     Calculate the number of ml/dose.
	6. 2 ml/dose

7. Ordered: Dolophine HCl 40 mg q4hr p.r.n.
     Available: Methadone HCl 10 mg/5 ml solution
     Calculate the number of tsp/dose.
	7. 4 tsp/dose

PROBLEM SET	PROBLEM SET ANSWERS

8. Ordered: Volmax 4 mg PO b.i.d.
   Available: Albuterol sulfate 2 mg/5 ml syrup
   Calculate the number of tsp/dose.

   8. 2 tsp/dose

9. Ordered: Colchicine 0.6 mg 2 tab PO, repeat q1hr until relief (max 9.6 mg/24 hr)
   Available: Colchicine 0.6-mg tab
   Calculate the maximum number of tab/24 hr.

   9. 16 tab/24 hr

10. Ordered: Aspirin 3.9 gm/d PO q.i.d.
    Available: Easprin 975-mg tab
    Calculate the number of tab/dose.

    10. 1 tab/dose

11. Ordered: Pentobarbital sodium 1.5 mg/kg per hr continuous IV infusion for your patient, who weighs 143 lb
    Available: Nembutal 50 mg/ml
    Calculate the number of ml of Nembutal for 24 hr continuous infusion.

    11. 46.8 ml/24 hr

12. Ordered: Phenobarbital 20 mg/kg at 50 mg/min for your patient, who weighs 197 lb
    Available: Phenobarbital 2000 mg in NS 100 ml.
    Calculate the flow rate in ml/hr.

    12. 150 ml/hr

$A \times O \times \text{Total \#} = \text{Ans}$

$A \times O \times \text{Total \#} \times U = \text{Ans}$

$A \times O \times \text{Total \#} \times U \times U = \text{Ans}$

Read the problem and the question carefully. You are being asked to count the number of children who will need the TB test.

A = single unit dose
O = 1 dose/child
D = total number of children = 166 doses
% = 75% = 75/100

$D \times \% = \text{Ans}$

Answer: The number of x-rays/year.

Total # = 9000 people
% = 12% reacted
= 12/100 reacted
% = 80% x-rayed
= 80/100 x-rayed

Total # × % × % = Ans

CORRECT setup:

1. vial/d:

$$\frac{\text{vial}}{10 \ \cancel{\text{ml}}} \times \frac{0.1 \ \cancel{\text{ml}}}{\cancel{\text{dose}}} \times \frac{80 \ \cancel{\text{doses}}}{\text{d}} = 0.8 = 1 \ \text{vial/d}$$

2. vial/wk:

$$\frac{\text{vial}}{10 \ \cancel{\text{ml}}} \times \frac{0.1 \ \cancel{\text{ml}}}{\cancel{\text{dose}}} \times \frac{80 \ \cancel{\text{doses}}}{\cancel{\text{d}}} \times \frac{6 \ \cancel{\text{d}}}{\text{wk}} = 4.8 = 5 \ \text{vials/wk}$$

3. vial/mo:

$$\frac{\text{vial}}{10 \ \cancel{\text{ml}}} \times \frac{0.1 \ \cancel{\text{ml}}}{\cancel{\text{dose}}} \times \frac{80 \ \cancel{\text{doses}}}{\cancel{\text{d}}} \times \frac{6 \ \cancel{\text{d}}}{\cancel{\text{wk}}} \times \frac{4 \ \cancel{\text{wk}}}{\text{mo}} = 19.2 = 20 \ \text{vials/mo}$$

EXAMPLE 2

The school district in a small town in the Midwest is planning to do a mass TB screening with the tine tests for all of their pupils enrolled in kindergarten (63), 7th grade (56), and 11th grade (47). They anticipate 75% of the children will be screened (with consent forms signed by a parent or guardian). How many tine tests will the school nurse need?

Pertinent information provided: Total number of children = 63 + 56 + 47 = 166 children; 75% attendance
Unit equivalency conversion: None needed
Desired unit: dose/tine test

CORRECT setup:

$$166 \ \text{doses} \times \frac{75}{100} = 124.5 = 125 \ \text{doses}$$

EXAMPLE 3

In one US city, 9000 people are screened for TB each year. The incidence of positive tests is 12%. These people now need chest x-rays. How many chest x-rays should be anticipated each year if 80% of the positive reactors get the x-rays?

M I N I   Q U I Z

What is the question asking you to solve?

Pertinent information provided: 9000 people/yr; 12% reacted; 80% x-rayed
Unit equivalency conversion: None needed
Desired unit: x-ray/yr

CORRECT setup:

$$\frac{9000 \ \cancel{\text{people}}}{\text{yr}} \times \frac{12 \ \cancel{\text{people reacted}}}{100 \ \cancel{\text{people}}} \times \frac{80 \ \text{people x-rayed}}{100 \ \cancel{\text{people reacted}}}$$

$$= 864 \ \text{people x-rayed/yr}$$

EXAMPLE   4

A group of 2267 children were screened for TB using the Mantoux test (0.1-ml test dose). Available is PPD 10-ml vials. Calculate the number of vials needed for this screening program.

Pertinent information provided: 2267 doses; 0.1 ml/dose; 10 ml/vial
Unit equivalency conversion: None needed
Desired unit: vial

CORRECT setup:

$$\frac{\text{vial}}{10 \text{ ml}} \times \frac{0.1 \text{ ml}}{\text{dose}} \times 2267 \text{ doses} = 22.67 = 23 \text{ vials}$$

Total # = 2267
children = 2267 doses

A × O × Total # = Ans

CALCULATIONS FOR DRUG ADMINISTRATION IN FLU AND PNEUMONIA VACCINE CLINICS FOR SENIORS AND OTHER HIGH-RISK POPULATIONS

Flu vaccinations are recommended once a year for all adults over the age of 65. A new flu vaccine formula is made up each year in anticipation of the suspected strain of flu that will be experienced during the winter. The pneumonia vaccine needs to be given only once. Some providers, however, recommend giving senior citizens the pneumonia vaccine every 6 years after age 65, because the immune response declines with age and the "booster" pneumonia vaccine is designed to provide added protection.

The Centers for Disease Control and Prevention (CDC) recommend that certain high-risk individuals should consider getting the yearly flu vaccine. Patients at risk include children and young adults with asthma, as well as anyone with a compromised health state or a debilitating illness. Patients at risk tend to be resistant or develop resistance to treatment modalities. In addition, they tend to have difficulty in recovering from the flu. Therefore, the CDC recommend the added precaution of a yearly dose of flu vaccine.

EXAMPLE   1

A city health department is mobilizing its efforts to have flu clinics available at 25 community senior centers by the fall. They are anticipating 13,500 attendees (0.5 ml/dose). Available is the flu vaccine multidose 10-ml vials.

1. How many vials will be needed?
2. Calculate the number of cartons of flu vaccine (12 vial/carton).
3. About 15% of the seniors will also be receiving the pneumonia vaccine (0.5 ml/dose). Available is the Pneumovax single-dose vial, 5-vial box. Calculate the number of boxes of pneumonia vaccine.

Pertinent information provided: 13,500 attendees; 0.5 ml/dose flu; 10 ml/vial flu; 15% Pneumovax; 5 doses/box Pneumovax
Unit equivalency conversion: None needed
Desired units: (1) vials of flu vaccine; (2) cartons of flu vaccine; (3) boxes of Pneumovax

This question has many components, so be sure to extract the pertinent information for each part.

Even though this question has many parts, it is a realistic situation for a public health nurse.

A = 10 ml/vial flu
A = single dose Pneumovax
A = 5 doses/box Pneumovax
O = 0.5 ml/dose (flu and pneumo)
% = 15% = 15/100
Total # = 13,500 people = 13,500 doses

A × O × Total # = Ans

A × Total # = Ans

A × % × Total # = Ans

Adult, age >12 yr, to receive 0.5-ml/dose; Children, age <3 yr, to receive 0.25 ml/dose.

A = 10 ml/vial
O = 0.5 ml/dose adult
= 0.25 ml/dose child
Total # = 500 adult
doses = 250 child doses

A × O × Total # = Ans

Adult + Children = Ans

A = 10 ml/vial
= 12 vials/carton
O = 0.5 ml/dose
Total # = 2,000,000
doses

A × A × O × Total # = Ans

CORRECT setup:

1. vials of flu vaccine:

$$\frac{\text{vial}}{10 \ \text{ml}} \times \frac{0.5 \ \text{ml}}{\text{dose}} \times 13{,}500 \ \text{doses} = 675 \ \text{vials}$$

2. cartons of flu vaccine:

$$\frac{\text{carton}}{12 \ \text{vials}} \times 675 \ \text{vials} = 56.25 = 57 \ \text{cartons of flu vaccine}$$

3. boxes of Pneumovax:

$$\frac{\text{box}}{5 \ \text{doses}} \times \frac{15}{100} \times 13{,}500 \ \text{doses} = 405 \ \text{boxes of Pneumovax}$$

E X A M P L E 2

An asthma society in a large city is recommending the flu vaccine for asthma sufferers of all ages. Members of the society are working with county community health nurses to offer six flu clinics in the fall. They are preparing for 500 adults (0.5 ml/dose) and 250 children (0.25 ml/dose) to attend. How many vials of flu vaccine will they need (10 ml/vials)?

Pertinent information provided: 0.5 ml/adult dose: 0.25 ml/child dose; 10 ml/vial

Unit equivalency conversion: None needed

Desired unit: vial

CORRECT setup:

$$\frac{\text{vial}}{10 \ \text{ml}} \times \frac{0.5 \ \text{ml}}{\text{dose}} \times 500 \ \text{doses} = 25 \ \text{vials}$$

$$\frac{\text{vial}}{10 \ \text{ml}} \times \frac{0.25 \ \text{ml}}{\text{dose}} \times 250 \ \text{doses} = 6.25 = 7 \ \text{vials}$$

Total number of vials = 25 + 7 = 32 vials of flu vaccine

E X A M P L E 3

A populous state is preparing to have an adequate supply of flu vaccine to meet statewide demands. The state is preparing to have enough vaccine to administer 2,000,000 doses of adult flu vaccine at 0.5 ml/dose. Available is multidose flu vaccine in 10-ml vials, with 12 vial/carton. Calculate the number of cartons for this campaign.

Pertinent information provided: 2,000,000 doses; 0.5 ml/dose; 10 ml/vial; 12 vials/carton

Unit equivalency conversion: None needed

Desired unit: carton

CORRECT setup:

$$\frac{\text{carton}}{12 \ \text{vials}} \times \frac{\text{vial}}{10 \ \text{ml}} \times \frac{0.5 \ \text{ml}}{\text{dose}} \times 2{,}000{,}000 \ \text{doses} = 8333.3 = 8334 \ \text{cartons}$$

EXAMPLE   4

All seven home health nurses in an agency are to administer the flu vaccine to clients (0.5-ml dose) over the age of 65 who will be visited during the month of October. If all of the clients in that age group give consent, how many vials (10-ml vial) of vaccine will the agency need to have available in October for the nurses who will be visiting a total of 234 clients? If each nurse visits ⅟₇ of the clients, how many vials will each nurse use?

Pertinent information provided: 234 doses/7 nurses; 0.5 ml/dose; 10 ml/vial

Unit equivalency conversion: None needed

Desired unit: vial

CORRECT setup:

$$\frac{vial}{10 \text{ ml}} \times \frac{0.5 \text{ ml}}{dose} \times \frac{234 \text{ doses}}{7 \text{ nurses}} = 1.7 = 2 \text{ vials/nurse}$$

A = 10 ml/vial
O = 0.5 ml/dose
Total # = 234 doses administered by seven nurses

A × O × Total # = Ans

Chapter Summary

The preceding examples highlight some of the typical vaccine and immunization needs of health care practitioners working in the community. The dosages focused on three areas: immunization of children, TB screening, and flu and pneumonia immunization programs for seniors and high-risk patients. Also, the current recommended immunization schedule for infants and children is provided in the Appendix.

Although the examples may appear convoluted and complex, they are easily simplified through the DA process. This chapter on using DA in the community is important because increasing numbers of nurses are working in the community as changes in our health care delivery system occur. You cannot leave your medication dosage calculations behind in the hospital. You will need to use them in the community as well.

If you have difficulty in following the examples presented in this chapter, it would be wise to review Chapters 4 and 5, because most immunizations and vaccines are ordered as oral and/or injectable doses. Again, you are reminded to research all medications that are unfamiliar to you prior to administering them to your patients. You will need to be prepared to explain side effects and adverse reactions to patients or those responsible for their care. Information on side effects or adverse reactions has not been presented in this chapter. This information can be found in any pharmacology textbook.

PROBLEM SET

1. How many pediatric doses of Flu-Immune (influenza purified surface antigen) are there in a 10-ml vial?

PROBLEM SET ANSWERS

1. 40 doses/vial

PROBLEM SET	PROBLEM SET ANSWERS
2. How many adult doses of Flu-Immune are there in 10-ml vial?	2. 20 doses/vial
3. If you are administering the DTP vaccine to 440 children, how many vials are needed?	3. 22 vials
4. If you are administering the diphtheria, tetanus, pertussis (DTP) vaccine to 440 children, and you have 12 vials in a carton, how many cartons do you need?	4. 2 cartons
5. If you are administering the DTP vaccine to 440 children, and you have 12 vials in a carton, will there be any vials left over?	5. Yes, 2 vials left over
6. Hep-B-Gammagee (hepatitis B immune globulin) 0.5 ml IM is ordered for 33 adults exposed to hepatitis B. You go to their work site to administer the vaccine. How many 10-ml vials will you need to have with you?	6. 2 vials
7. Nationally, 29,000,000 adults receive the flu vaccine each year. Calculate the number of 10-ml vials that are needed annually.	7. 1,450,000 vials

PROBLEM SET	PROBLEM SET ANSWERS

8. Nationally 29,000,000 adults receive the flu vaccine each year. Calculate the number of cartons (12 vials/carton) used.

   8. 120,833.3 = 120,834 cartons

9. If there are 100 adult doses (0.5 ml/dose) of flu vaccine in five vials, how many pediatric doses (0.25 ml/dose) are there?

   9. 200 doses

10. A school system is conducting TB screening of its 456 employees, using the Mantoux test (0.1 ml/dose). How many 10-ml vials does the school system need?

   10. 4.56 = 5 vials

11. In TB screening of 456 employees with the Mantoux test, if each vial contains 2 ml, how many vials are needed?

   11. 22.8 = 23 vials

12. The measles, mumps, and rubella (MMR) vaccine is administered twice (at age 1 and between ages 4 and 6) as part of the recommended childhood immunization schedule. A clinic is preparing to administer MMR immunizations to infants and children. They expect to administer the vaccine to 350 children in 1 mo. How many 10-ml vials will be needed?

   12. 17.5 = 18 vials

PROBLEM SET	PROBLEM SET ANSWERS
13. A large state health department is preparing a list of the amount of DTP vaccines needed for the year. They will need 7,500,000 doses of DTP. Available is DTP toxoid 0.5 ml/dose in 10-ml vials. a. How many 10-ml vials of DTP will be needed?	13. a. 375,000 10-ml vials of DTP
b. How many 12-vial cartons of DTP will be needed?	b. 31,250 12-vial cartons of DTP
14. The same state health department estimated 5,000,000 doses of MMR vaccines for the year. Available is MMR vaccine in single-dose vials (reconstituted with diluent to 0.5 ml/dose), 20 vials/box. Calculate the number of boxes of single-dose vials with 20 vials/box.	14. MMR: 250,000 boxes
15. There are six cartons (10 ml/vial) of 12 vials each of flu vaccine in a city health department. Calculate the number of available adult (0.5 ml/dose) doses.	15. 1440 adult doses
16. There are six cartons (10 ml/vial) of 12 vials each of flu vaccine in a city health department. Calculate the number of pediatric doses (0.25 ml/dose).	16. 2880 pediatric doses

PROBLEM SET	PROBLEM SET ANSWERS
17. Children of preschool and kindergarten age require a booster of DTP (acellular) (0.5 ml/dose) and poliovirus vaccines. A rural clinic estimates that approximately 150 children will be registering to enter preschool and kindergarten classes. Available is Infanrix (DTaP) in 10-ml vials. Calculate the number of vials of DTaP that the clinic will need to request through the free vaccine program.	17. $7.5 = 8$ vials
18. Children of preschool and kindergarten age require a booster of DTP (acellular) (0.5 ml/dose) and poliovirus vaccines. A rural clinic estimates that approximately 150 children will be registering to enter preschool and kindergarten classes. Calculate the number of packages of Orimune (poliovirus vaccine, live oral trivalent) single-dose units in 10 units per package.	18. 15 packages
19. Children of preschool and kindergarten age require boosters of DTP (acellular) (0.5 ml/dose) and poliovirus vaccines. A rural clinic estimates that approximately 150 children will be registering to enter preschool and kindergarten classes. Calculate the number of packages of Orimune single-dose units in 50 units per package.	19. 3 packages
20. Of the 250 children who will need an oral polio vaccine, a rural health clinic has estimated that approximately 10% would opt for the inactivated poliovirus vaccine (IPV). Calculate the number of packages of 10 single-dose units per package.	20. $2.5 = 3$ packages

PROBLEM SET	PROBLEM SET ANSWERS
21. Of the 8560 people screened for TB in one city, 5% tested positive and needed follow-up chest x-rays. Calculate the number of people who would need the x-rays.	21. 428 people needed chest x-rays
22. A student health center located on a college campus estimates that 50% of the freshman students will require MMR (0.5 ml/dose) and tetanus-diphtheria toxoid (Td) (0.5 ml/dose) boosters. The enrollment at the beginning of the academic year is 1058 students. Calculate the number of vials of multidose MMR and Td 10-ml/vial, 12 vials/carton.	22. 27 vials of each MMR and Td
23. A student health center located on a college campus estimates that 50% of the freshman students will require MMR (0.5 ml/dose) and Td (0.5 ml/dose) boosters. The enrollment at the beginning of the academic year is 1058 students. Calculate the number of cartons of MMR and Td 10 ml/vial, 12 vials/carton.	23. 3 cartons of MMR and 3 cartons of Td
24. A student health center located on a college campus estimates that 50% of the freshman students will require MMR (0.5 ml/dose) and Td (0.5 ml/dose) boosters. The enrollment at the beginning of the academic year is 1058 students. The health center estimates that 80% of the students will require Hep-B-Gammagee (HepB) vaccine (3 doses/student over a period of 6 mo). Calculate the number of cartons of HepB vaccine (0.5 ml/dose), 10-ml vials and 12 vials/carton, for the year's freshmen.	24. 10.6 = 11 cartons

Some Facts About Medication Calculations With Large Groups of People

1. Flu vaccine can be drawn up in advance (24 hr) if kept refrigerated.
2. A well child can receive more than one immunization at one time.
3. Even if a child has a minor cold, the immunization can usually be given in order to avoid a "missed opportunity."
4. Prior to the administration of immunizations, it is important to obtain a signed consent form from the adult patient, parent or guardian of a minor child.
5. The three rights and the five checks must be carried out prior to the administration of medications or vaccines.
6. As part of the nursing process, instruct patients about potential side and adverse effects.
7. A child's parents or guardians have the right to refuse all childhood immunizations.
8. The lot number, manufacturer of the vaccine, and site of administration must be documented after the administration of an immunization.
9. Prior to administration, study the drug information that comes with the multiple-dose vial of vaccine and to check for side effects and adverse drug reactions.
10. Flu vaccines are administered to adults who have completed an informed consent form and received information about side effects and possible adverse reactions prior to administration.
11. You must always orient your desired dimension in the proper numerator/denominator positions in the DA setup.
12. The flu and pneumonia vaccines can be administered at the same time.
13. The flu vaccine is given yearly; however, certain high-risk populations may receive the flu vaccine twice a year.
14. The pneumonia vaccine is usually given only once, but it cannot be given more often than every 6 years.
15. Place firm pressure over the site of an IM injection after administration.
16. Oral poliovirus and chickenpox virus vaccines must be kept frozen until the time of administration.
17. The chickenpox virus vaccine must be reconstituted and used within 30 min.
18. Vaccines requiring SC administration should not be administered IM.
19. The deltoid and gluteal muscles are not sufficiently developed to be used as injection sites in pediatric patients under 2 years of age.

[12]

Populations Needing Special Therapies: Medication Calculation Considerations Using Dimensional Analysis

INTRODUCTION

This chapter demonstrates dosage calculation for the administration of medications to populations needing special therapies or settings. The scenario that accompanies each dosage problem describes a unique situation. Dosages that are administered cyclically and/or over a significant length of time will be presented, for example, beyond the average schedule of 7 to 10 d. Additionally, medications are included with dosing schedules that change rapidly, depending on the patient's response, for example, dosages used in advanced cardiac life-support algorithms.

Despite the increasing complexity of medication orders, you will see that the process of calculation is similar to that demonstrated in previous chapters. By categorizing information provided in each question into pertinent and irrelevant facts, you can apply dimensional analysis (DA) in solving the problem without needing to recall specific formulas. As in previous chapters, you simply use information provided in the problem (as well as the unit equivalency tables found in the Appendix) as conversion factors, and place them in the proper numerator/denominator orientation for unit cancellation.

Scenarios have been prepared from various areas to acquaint students with dosage administration in different aspects of nursing.

LEARNING OBJECTIVES

By the end of this chapter, you will be able to calculate medication dosages for patients in need of:

- Chemotherapy

- Poison management

- Maintenance of hemodynamic support

CALCULATIONS FOR DRUG ADMINISTRATION OF CHEMOTHERAPEUTIC AGENTS

Chemotherapeutic agents are administered in either inpatient or outpatient settings. The ready availability of numerous medications that adequately control gastrointestinal adverse effects has helped to increase use of chemotherapy administration in outpatient settings.

The following examples demonstrate dosage calculation for administration of chemotherapeutic agents.

Cyclic administration of highly cytotoxic medications, such as chemotherapeutic agents, often necessitates the placement of a catheter for central venous or arterial access, that is, a central line.

Ord = 12 mg/kg per dose

E X A M P L E   1

Adrucil 12 mg/kg over 24 hr for 4 d, pause 3 d, repeat cycle for treatment of colon cancer, is ordered for your patient, who weighs 154 lb. Available is fluorouracil 500 mg/10 ml. Calculate the number of ml/dose.

Pertinent information provided: 12 mg/kg; 154 lb; 500 mg/10 ml
Unit equivalency conversion: 2.2 lb/kg
Desired unit: ml/dose

CORRECT setup:

$$\frac{12 \text{ mg}}{\text{kg} \cdot \text{dose}} \times \frac{10 \text{ ml}}{500 \text{ mg}} \times \frac{\text{kg}}{2.2 \text{ lb}} \times 154 \text{ lb} = 16.8 \text{ ml/dose}$$

Implement the five rights and the three checks before administration of medication to your patients.

Ord × A × U × BW = Ans

E X A M P L E   2

Cytoxan 10 mg/kg in 100 ml D_5W IVPB q.d. for 10 d is ordered as part of the combination therapy for treatment of lupus in your patient, who weighs 144 lb. Available is lyophilized cyclophosphamide reconstituted to 20 mg/ml. Calculate the number of ml/dose.

Ord = 10 mg/kg per dose over 10 d

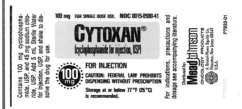

Chemotherapeutic agents are frequently reconstituted and/or diluted by the pharmacist and delivered to you for administration.

Pertinent information provided: 10 mg/kg; 144 lb; 20 mg/ml
Unit equivalency conversion: 2.2 lb/kg
Desired unit: ml/dose

CORRECT setup:

$$\frac{10 \text{ mg}}{\text{kg} \cdot \text{dose}} \times \frac{\text{ml}}{20 \text{ mg}} \times \frac{\text{kg}}{2.2 \text{ lb}} \times 144 \text{ lb} = 32.7 \text{ ml/dose}$$

Ord × A × U × BW = Ans

E X A M P L E   3

Doxorubicin HCl 75 mg/m² per d IVPB every 21 d is ordered for the treatment of breast cancer in your patient, who weighs 178 lb and is 5′6″ tall. Available is Adriamycin 2 mg/ml in 50-ml vials. Calculate the number of mg/d.

BSA from nomogram for 178 lb, 5′6″ = 1.95 m²
Ord = 75 mg/m² per d

M I N I   Q U I Z

Name the five rights.

Pertinent information provided: 75 mg/m² per d; 178 lb; 5′6″
Unit equivalency conversion: BSA from the nomogram (see Appendix)
Desired unit: mg/d

CORRECT setup:

$$\frac{75 \text{ mg}}{\text{m}^2 \cdot \text{d}} \times 1.95 \text{ m}^2 = 146.25 \text{ mg/d}$$

The abbreviation for feet = ft. The symbol to abbreviate ft = ′. The abbreviation for inch = in. The symbol to abbreviate in = ″.

Ord × BSA = Ans

E X A M P L E   4

VePesid 35 mg/m² per d IVPB at 200 μg/ml of NS concentration over 60 min q.o.d. for 5 d qwk for 4 wk is ordered for the treatment of small cell carcinoma of the lung in your patient, who weighs 112 lb, and is 4′6″ tall. Available is etoposide for injection in 500 mg/25 ml vials.

BSA from nomogram for 112 lb, 4′ 6″. = 1.35 m²
Ord = 35 mg/m² per d
DF = 15 gtt/ml
Oc = 200 μg/ml
Ot = 60 min

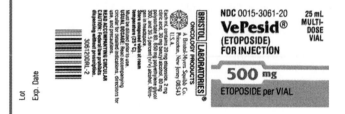

1. Calculate the number of mg/dose.
2. Calculate the total volume for infusion.
3. Calculate the drip rate in gtt/min (15 gtt/ml).

Pertinent information provided: 35 mg/m² per d; 112 lb; 4′6″;
    200 μg/ml; 15 gtt/ml; 500 mg/25 ml.
Unit equivalency conversion: BSA from nomogram; 1000 μg/mg
Desired units: (1) mg/dose; (2) total volume/dose; (3) gtt/min

CORRECT setup:

1. mg/dose:

$$\frac{35 \text{ mg}}{\text{m}^2 \cdot \text{d}} \times 1.35 \text{ m}^2 = 47.25 \text{ mg/dose}$$

Ord × BSA = Ans

2. total volume:

$$\frac{\text{ml}}{200 \text{ μg}} \times \frac{1000 \text{ μg}}{\text{mg}} \times \frac{47.25 \text{ mg}}{\text{dose}} = 236.25 = 236 \text{ ml dose}$$

Oc × U × O = Ans

$$\frac{25 \text{ ml}}{500 \text{ mg}} \times \frac{35 \text{ mg}}{\text{m}^2 \cdot \text{d}} \times 1.35 \text{ m}^2 = 2.36 \text{ ml VePesid}$$

You will start with an NS 250-ml unit bag and use a syringe to draw out 12 ml, leaving 238 ml in the bag. Then add 2.36 ml VePesid.

Drip factor (DF) × Ov ×
Ot = Ans

BSA from the nomogram
for 142 lb, 5′11″ =
1.83 m²
Ord = 200 mg/m² per d
Oc = 1 mg/ml
Ot = 24 hr

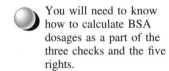

You will need to know
how to calculate BSA
dosages as a part of the
three checks and the five
rights.

Ord × BSA = Ans

Ov × Ot = Ans

BSA from nomogram for
164 lb, 5′8″ = 1.9 m²
Ord = 3.3 mg/m² per d
Ot = 4 hr

---

3. gtt/min:

$$\frac{15 \text{ gtt}}{\text{ml}} \times \frac{236 \text{ ml}}{\text{dose}} \times \frac{\text{dose}}{60 \text{ min}} = 59 \text{ gtt/min}$$

E X A M P L E   5

Platinol 200 mg/m² per d IVPB at 1 mg/ml concentration over 24 hr for 5 d, repeat q3wk, is ordered for treatment of ovarian carcinoma in your patient, who weighs 142 lb, and is 5′11″ tall. Available is cisplatin for reconstitution in 100 mg/100 ml vials for injection.

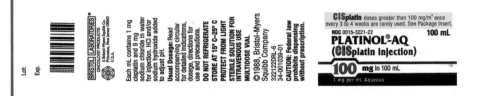

1. Calculate the number of mg of cisplatin/d.
2. Calculate the flow rate in ml/hr.

Pertinent information provided: 200 mg/m² per d; 142 lb; 5′11″
Unit equivalency conversion: BSA from the nomogram
Desired units: (1) mg/dose; (2) ml/hr

CORRECT setup:

1. mg/dose:

$$\frac{200 \text{ mg}}{\text{m}^2 \cdot \text{d}} \times 1.83 \text{ m}^2 = 366 \text{ mg/d (dose)}$$

2. ml/hr:

$$\frac{366 \text{ ml}}{\text{dose}} \times \frac{\text{dose}}{24 \text{ hr}} = 15.25 = 15 \text{ ml/hr}$$

E X A M P L E   6

Methotrexate sodium 3.3 mg/m² per d IVPB with 100 ml of D₅W concentration over 4 hr is ordered for the treatment of lymphocytic leukemia in your patient, who weighs 164 lb and is 5′8″ tall. Available is methotrexate sodium injection, 25 mg/ml.

1. Calculate the number of mg of methotrexate sodium/d.
2. Calculate the flow rate in ml/hr.

Pertinent information provided: 3.3 mg/m² per d; 25 mg/ml; 164 lb; 5′8″; 100 ml/dose
Unit equivalency conversion: BSA from the nomogram
Desired units: (1) ml/dose; (2) ml/hr

CORRECT setup:

1. ml methotrexate:

$$\frac{\text{ml}}{25 \text{ mg}} \times \frac{3.3 \text{ mg}}{\text{m}^2 \cdot \text{d}} \times 1.9 \text{ m}^2 = 0.25 \text{ ml/dose}$$

A × Ord × BSA = Ans

2. flow rate (ml/hr):

$$\frac{100 \text{ ml}}{\text{dose}} \times \frac{\text{dose}}{4 \text{ hr}} = 25 \text{ ml/hr}$$

DF × Ov × Ot = Ans

E X A M P L E   7

Taxol 135 mg/m² per dose IVPB at 0.3 mg/ml concentration diluted with D₅W, given over 24 hr every 21 d, is ordered for the treatment of ovarian cancer in your patient, who weighs 127 lb and is 5′5″ tall. Available are vials of paclitaxel for injection at a dose of 30 mg/5 ml.

BSA from the nomogram for 127 lb, 5′5″ = 1.63 m²
Ord = 135 mg/m² per d
Oc = 0.3 mg/ml
Ot = 24 hr

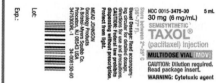

1. Calculate the number of ml of Taxol/dose.
2. Calculate the total volume for infusion.
3. Calculate the flow rate in ml/hr.

Know the trade and generic names of the medications you administer.

   Pertinent information provided: 135 mg/m² per d; 30 mg/5 ml; 127 lb; 5′5″; 0.3 mg/ml
   Unit equivalency conversion: BSA from the nomogram
   Desired units: (1) ml/dose; (2) ml diluent/dose; (3) ml/hr

CORRECT setup:

1. ml/dose:

$$\frac{5 \text{ ml}}{30 \text{ mg}} \times \frac{135 \text{ mg}}{\text{m}^2 \cdot \text{d}} \times 1.63 \text{ m}^2 = 36.7 \text{ ml/dose}$$

Ord × A × BSA = Ans

2. Total volume/dose:

$$\frac{135 \text{ mg}}{\text{m}^2 \cdot \text{dose}} \times 163 \text{ m}^2 = 220.05 \text{ mg/dose}$$

Oc × O = Ans

$$\frac{\text{ml}}{0.3 \text{ mg}} \times \frac{220.05 \text{ mg}}{\text{dose}} = 733.5 = 734 \text{ ml/dose}$$

Start with two 500-ml D₅W unit bags and, using a 30-ml syringe, draw 200 ml from one and inject it into the other plus 36.7 ml Taxol to total 734 ml.

Total volume = Taxol + Diluent

3. ml/hr:

$$\frac{734 \text{ ml}}{\text{dose}} \times \frac{\text{dose}}{24 \text{ hr}} = 30.6 = 31 \text{ ml/hr}$$

Ov × U × Ot = Ans

CALCULATIONS FOR DRUG ADMINISTRATION IN POISON MANAGEMENT

The administration of medication dosages in poison management is normally carried out in the emergency department. Medication administration is carried out rapidly, because time is of the essence, especially when you are treating acutely ill patients.

The following are examples of medication dosage calculations that could typically appear on orders for treating patients who have ingested or injected poisons.

In the emergency setting, you are likely to be working as a team member to accommodate the patient's medication and/or procedural needs.

E X A M P L E   1

To induce emesis, syrup of ipecac 30 ml PO stat is ordered for your patient who was brought to the emergency department after ingestion of a noncorrosive poison. Available is a 15 ml/unit dose of ipecac syrup, USP. Calculate the number of units per dose.

Pertinent information provided: 30 ml/dose; 15 ml/unit
Unit equivalency conversion: None needed
Desired unit: unit/dose

Have a container ready to catch the emesis.

Use a poison chart to determine if vomiting is indicated.

CORRECT setup:

$$\frac{unit}{15\ \text{ml}} \times \frac{30\ \text{ml}}{dose} = 2\ unit/dose$$

$$A \quad \times \quad O \quad = \quad Ans$$

Vomiting should be induced *only* if the substance is noncorrosive.
- If substances such as lye, bleach, or corrosives are vomited, they will damage the gastrointestinal tract a second time.
- A petroleum product causes aspiration if vomiting is induced.

NDC 0054-8425   **DELIVERS 15 mL/OFRECE 15 mL**   EXP. LOT

IPECAC SYRUP USP

EMETIC   Alcohol 1.75%
For emergency use to cause vomiting of swallowed poisons. See Carton Label. Usual dosage: Adults and children 12 yrs and over – 30 mL; children 1 to under 12 yrs – 15 mL; children 6 mo to under 1 yr – 5 mL; followed by a large quantity of water.   4215500   054

FOR ORAL USE   Roxane Laboratories

EMETICO   Alcohol 1.75%
Para usar en caso de emergencia para provocar el vómito de venenos ingeridos. Vea la etiqueta en el cartón. Dosis usual: Adultos y niños de 12 años y mayores – 30 mL; niños de 1 a menores de 12 años – 15 mL; niños de 6 meses a menores de 1 año – 5 mL; acompañado de una gran cantidad de aqua.

Columbus, OH 43216 PARA USO ORAL

E X A M P L E   2

Gastric lavage tap water 15 ml/kg is ordered for a patient who was admitted to the emergency department for ingestion of a toxic dose of Nembutal Sodium. The patient weighs 174 lb. Calculate the number of ml of tap water needed to carry out a gastric lavage with an orogastric tube.

Pertinent information provided: 15 ml/kg; 174 lb
Unit equivalency conversion: 2.2 lb/kg
Desired unit: ml/dose

To decrease aspiration, place the patient in the Trendelenburg, left lateral decubitus position.

Ord = 15 ml/kg

Ord × U × BW = Ans

CORRECT setup:

$$\frac{15\ ml}{\text{kg}} \times \frac{\text{kg}}{2.2\ \text{lb}} \times 174\ \text{lb} = 1186\ ml/dose$$

EXAMPLE 3

The reference dose for an activated charcoal suspension is 1 to 2 gm/kg per 8 ml of fluid (tap water with a flavoring agent). The patient weighs 158 lb. Available is Liqui-Char in 50-gm units.

1. Calculate the number of gm/dose of charcoal,
2. Calculate the number of fl oz needed for mixing.

Pertinent information provided: 1 to 2 gm/kg; 158 lb; 8 ml fluid/dose of 1 to 2 gm
Unit equivalency conversion: 2.2 lb/kg
Desired units: (1) gm/dose; (2) fl oz/dose

 A premixed formula of activated charcoal is available as Actidose in 15-, 25-, and 50-gm unit doses. Mix the charcoal with the smallest amount of fluid to administer the dosage rapidly, that is, in one or two gulps.

CORRECT setup:

1. gm/dose charcoal:

$$\frac{1 \text{ to } 2 \text{ gm}}{\cancel{kg}} \times \frac{\cancel{kg}}{2.2 \text{ \cancel{lb}}} \times 158 \text{ \cancel{lb}} = 72 \text{ to } 144 \text{ gm/dose}$$

 Ord Charcoal = 1 to 2 gm/kg
Fluid for mixing = 8 ml/2 gm

2. fl oz/dose:

$$\frac{8 \text{ \cancel{ml}}}{1 \text{ to } 2 \text{ \cancel{gm}}} \times \frac{72 \text{ to } 144 \text{ \cancel{gm}}}{\text{dose}} \times \frac{\text{fl oz}}{30 \text{ \cancel{ml}}} = 9.6 \text{ to } 19.2 \text{ fl oz/dose}$$

 Ord × U × BW = Ans

 Ord × O × U = Ans

In reality, you will use the smallest possible amount of water to suspend the charcoal, because the more water you use in the mixture, the more the patient will have to drink to receive the ordered dose (up to 19 fl oz).

To administer, mix the charcoal with 10 fl oz of water.

 If necessary, you can always add more water.

EXAMPLE 4

Whole-bowel irrigation with 4 L of polyethylene glycol and electrolytes over 3 hr, via nasogastric tube, is ordered for a patient who has ingested a toxic amount of iron sulfate ($FeSO_4$). Available is a 4-L container of GoLYTELY. Calculate the flow rate in ml/hr.
Pertinent information provided: 4 L/dose; 3 hr/dose
Unit equivalency conversion: 1000 ml/L
Desired unit: ml/hr

 Reconstitute GoLYTELY in the container, using lukewarm water that is filled to the mark. Shake the container until the powder is dissolved

CORRECT setup:

$$\frac{1000 \text{ ml}}{\cancel{L}} \times \frac{4 \text{ \cancel{L}}}{\cancel{dose}} \times \frac{\cancel{dose}}{3 \text{ hr}} = 1333.33 \text{ ml} = 1333 \text{ ml/hr}$$

 Ov = 4 L
Ot = 3 hr

 U × Ov × Ot = Ans
Round numbers to the nearest measurable unit.

EXAMPLE 5

Phytonadione 10 mg IVPB over 60 min is ordered as a part of treating salicylate poisoning. Available is AquaMEPHYTON 10 mg in 100 ml of D_5W. Calculate the drip rate in gtt/min (15 gtt/ml).
Pertinent information provided: 100 ml/dose; 60 min/dose; 15 gtt/ml
Unit equivalency conversion: None needed
Desired unit: gtt/min

 DF = 15 gtt/ml
Ov = 100 ml
Ot = 60 min

DF × Ov × Ot = Ans

 Ord = 2.5 mg/kg

 Check whether the patient is allergic to peanuts.

 A × Ord × U × BW = Ans
Round 2.125 ml to the nearest measurable unit of 2.1 ml. You will need only 2.1 ml of the 3-ml ampule.

 Total dose/regimen = (q.i.d. × 2 d) + (b.i.d. × 1 d) + (q.d. × 10 d) = Ans

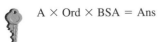 O × A × O = Ans

 BSA from the nomogram for 5′ and 51 kg = 1.49 m²
Ord = 1000 mg/m²

A × Ord × BSA = Ans

CORRECT setup:

$$\frac{15 \text{ gtt}}{\text{ml}} \times \frac{100 \text{ ml}}{\text{dose}} \times \frac{\text{dose}}{60 \text{ min}} = 25 \text{ gtt/min}$$

E X A M P L E   6

Dimercaprol in peanut oil 2.5 mg/kg IM q6hr for 2 d, then b.i.d. for 1 d, then q.d. for 10 d, is ordered to treat arsenic poisoning for a patient who weighs 187 lb. Available is BAL in Oil in 3-ml ampules of 100 mg/ml.

1. Calculate the number of ml/dose.
2. How many ampules would you need per dose?
3. How many ampules are needed for the regimen ordered?

Pertinent information provided: 2.5 mg/kg; 187 lb; 100 mg/ml; 3 ml/ampule; 4 dose/d for 2 d; 2 dose/d for 1 d; 1 dose/d for 10 d
Unit equivalency conversion: 2.2 lb/kg
Desired units: (1) ml/dose; (2) ampule/dose; (3) ampule/regimen

CORRECT setup:

1. ml/dose:

$$\frac{\text{ml}}{100 \text{ mg}} \times \frac{2.5 \text{ mg}}{\text{kg} \cdot \text{dose}} \times \frac{\text{kg}}{2.2 \text{ lb}} \times 187 \text{ lb} = 2.125 = 2.1 \text{ ml/dose}$$

2. One ampule will be sufficient for each dose.
3. ampule/regimen:

$$\frac{4 \text{ doses}}{\text{d}} \times 2 \text{ d} = 8 \text{ doses} + \left(\frac{2 \text{ doses}}{\text{d}} \times 1 \text{ d}\right) + \left(\frac{1 \text{ dose}}{\text{d}} \times 10 \text{ d}\right)$$
$$= 20 \text{ doses needed for the regimen}$$

$$\frac{2.1 \text{ ml}}{\text{dose}} \times \frac{\text{ampule}}{3 \text{ ml}} \times \frac{20 \text{ doses}}{\text{regimen}} = 14 \text{ ampule/regimen}$$

May need up to (4 × 2) + 2 + 10 = 20 ampules if medication cannot be drawn ahead of time.

E X A M P L E   7

Calcium Disodium Versenate 1000 mg/m² over 24 hr is ordered for your patient, who weighs 51 kg and is 5′ tall. Available are 5-ml ampules of edetate calcium disodium injection 200 mg/ml. Calculate the number of ml/dose. How many ampules will you need for this order?

Pertinent information provided: 1000 mg/m²; 51 kg; 5 ft; 200 mg/ml
Unit equivalency conversion: BSA from the nomogram
Desired unit: ml/dose

CORRECT setup:

$$\frac{\text{ml}}{200 \text{ mg}} \times \frac{1000 \text{ mg}}{\text{m}^2 \cdot \text{dose}} \times 1.49 \text{ m}^2 = 7.45 \text{ ml/dose}$$

Two ampules will be needed for this order.

EXAMPLE 8

Antivenin 150 ml in 500 ml NS IVPB over a 2 hr, and repeat q2hr, is ordered for the treatment of a venomous snakebite. Available are 10-ml vials of antivenin for immediate use after reconstitution. Calculate the number of vial per dose.

Pertinent information provided: 150 ml/dose; 10 ml/vial
Unit equivalency conversion: None needed
Desired unit: vial/dose

CORRECT setup:

$$\frac{\text{vial}}{10\ \text{ml}} \times \frac{150\ \text{ml}}{\text{dose}} = 15\ \text{vial/dose}$$

Antivenins contains horse serum globulins. Patients allergic to horse serum globulins will need additional interventions.

A × O = Ans

EXAMPLE 9

Mucomyst 10% solution at 140 mg/kg loading dose, then 70 mg/kg q4hr for 17 doses, is ordered for acetaminophen ingestion. Your patient is 4 years old and weighs 38 lb. Your patient drank 4 fl oz of Tylenol 160 mg/5 ml. Available is acetylcysteine sodium 10% solution in a unit dose of 1 fl oz.

1. Calculate the number of fl oz for the loading dose.
2. Calculate the number of ml/dose for subsequent doses.

Pertinent information provided: 140 mg/kg; 70 mg/kg; 38 lb; 10% = 10 gm/100 ml; 1 fl oz/unit
Unit equivalency conversion: 2.2 lb/kg; 1000 mg/gm
Desired unit: fl oz/dose (loading and subsequent)

CORRECT setup:

1. fl oz/loading dose:

$$\frac{\text{fl oz}}{30\ \text{ml}} \times \frac{100\ \text{ml}}{10\ \text{gm}} \times \frac{\text{gm}}{1000\ \text{mg}} \times \frac{140\ \text{mg}}{\text{kg} \cdot \text{dose}} \times \frac{\text{kg}}{2.2\ \text{lb}} \times 38\ \text{lb} =$$

$$0.806 = 0.81\ \text{fl oz/loading dose}$$

It would be better to administer this order in ml: 24.18 = 24.2 ml/dose (30 ml = 1 fl oz)

2. fl oz/dose of subsequent doses:

70 mg/kg per dose = ½ loading dose or 0.403, rounded to 0.4 fl oz, or 12.1 ml/dose.

10% solution = 10 gm/100 ml

Ord = 140 mg/kg loading dose
Ord = 70 mg/kg subsequent dose

A × U × Ord × U × BW = Ans

The subsequent dose is one half of the loading dose.

EXAMPLE 10

Mucomyst 5%, administer 50 ml PO is ordered. Available is Mucomyst 20% in a 30-ml unit dose.

Review Chapter 4 if you have problems calculating the dosage dilutions.

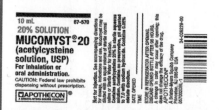

Oc = 5 gm/100 ml
Ac = 20 gm/100 ml
Ov = 50 ml

1. Calculate the number of ml of Mucomyst (20%) needed for this order.
2. How much tap water will you need to add for dilution?

Pertinent information provided: 5% = 5 gm/100 ml; 50 ml/dose of 5%; 20% = 20 gm/100 ml stock
Unit equivalency conversion: None needed
Desired unit: ml/dose Mucomyst 20%

CORRECT setup:

1. ml/dose Mucomyst:

Oc × Ov × A = Ans

$$\frac{5\ \text{gm}}{100\ \text{ml}\ (5\%)} \times \frac{50\ \text{ml}}{\text{dose}} \times \frac{100\ \text{ml}\ (20\%)}{20\ \text{gm}} = 12.5\ \text{ml/dose}$$

2. amount of tap water:

ml of tap water = 50 ml − 12.5 ml = 37.5 ml water/dose

Total volume − Mucomyst volume = Ans

CALCULATIONS FOR ADMINISTRATION OF HEMODYNAMIC SUPPORT

In this section, we will look at calculation of dosages for the administration of common medications used for cardiac life support, and other medications frequently administered in emergency and intensive care settings.

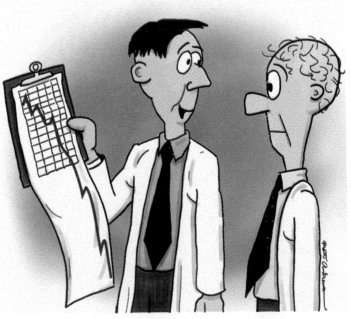

Medications administered for cardiac and circulatory support and/or resuscitation require constant cardiac monitoring.

"IT LOOKS LIKE MRS. STEVENS IS RESPONDING SPLENDIDLY TO HER NEW MEDICATION!"

EXAMPLE 1

Corvert 1 mg over 10 min IVSP is ordered for the treatment of atrial flutter. Available is Corvert (ibutilide fumarate) in vials of 1 mg/ml. Calculate the number of ml/min.

Pertinent information provided: 1 mg/10 min; 1 mg/ml
Unit equivalency conversion: None needed
Desired unit: ml/min

CORRECT setup:

$$\frac{ml}{1\ \cancel{mg}} \times \frac{1\ \cancel{mg}}{10\ min} = 0.1\ ml/min$$

 Or = 1 mg/10 min

 A × Or = Ans

EXAMPLE 2

Cardizem 20 mg IVSP over 10 min is ordered for your patient's atrial fibrillation. Available are Lyo-Ject Syringes of Cardizem (diltiazem HCl) 25 mg/5 ml. Calculate the number of ml/min.

Pertinent information provided: 20 mg/dose; 10 min/dose; 25 mg/5 ml
Unit equivalency conversion: None needed
Desired unit: ml/min

CORRECT setup:

$$\frac{5\ ml}{25\ \cancel{mg}} \times \frac{\cancel{dose}}{10\ min} \times \frac{20\ \cancel{mg}}{\cancel{dose}} = 0.4\ ml/min$$

 Ordered time (Ot) = 10 min/dose

 Lyo-Ject is a syringe with a screw-type plunger that eliminates the over- or underdosing of medication caused by friction between the plunger and the barrel.

 A × Ot × O = Ans

EXAMPLE 3

Epinephrine 2 mg in NS, a total volume of 10 ml via ET tube q3–5 min is the ACLS reference dose for ventricular fibrillation (Vfib) or pulseless ventricular tachycardia (Vtach). Available is epinephrine 1 mg/ml in vials of 30 ml. Calculate the number of ml epinephrine/dose.

Pertinent information provided: 2 mg/dose diluted to 10 ml NS
Unit equivalency conversion: None needed
Desired unit: ml/dose

CORRECT setup:

$$\frac{ml}{\cancel{mg}} \times \frac{2\ \cancel{mg}}{dose} = 2\ ml/dose$$

 You can draw up this order in the same way insulin mixtures are drawn. Inject air into the epinephrine and then the NS. Draw 8 ml of NS and then 2 ml of epinephrine.

 A × O = Ans

EXAMPLE 4

Bretylium tosylate 10 mg/kg, administered as an IV bolus q5–10min to a max of 30 mg/kg, is the ACLS reference dose for unresponsive Vfib and pulseless Vtach.

Available are prefilled syringes of bretylium tosylate 1 gm/20 ml. The patient weighs 295 lb. Calculate the number of ml/dose. How many doses can be administered to this patient?

Pertinent information provided: 10 mg/kg; 295 lb; 1 gm/20 ml; 30 mg/kg
Unit equivalency conversion: 2.2 lb/kg; 1000 mg/gm
Desired unit: ml/dose

 Ord = 10 mg/kg (30 mg/kg maximum)

 You can shorten the number of conversion factors in a continuous chain setup by first calculating the unit equivalency conversions, for example, lb to kg, gm to mg.

$A \times Ord \times U \times U \times BW = Ans$

CORRECT setup:

$$\frac{20 \text{ ml}}{1 \text{ gm}} \times \frac{10 \text{ mg}}{\text{kg}} \times \frac{1 \text{ gm}}{1000 \text{ mg}} \times \frac{\text{kg}}{2.2 \text{ lb}} \times 295 \text{ lb} = 26.8 \text{ ml/dose}$$

Maximum number of doses: 3 doses

$$\frac{\text{kg} \cdot \text{dose}}{10 \text{ mg}} \times \frac{30 \text{ mg}}{\text{kg}} = 3 \text{ doses}$$

E X A M P L E   5

Intropin 2.5 μg/kg per min continuous IV infusion is ordered for your patient, who weighs 102 lb. Available is dopamine HCl 200 mg in 250 ml of NS.

1. Calculate the number of gtt/min (15 gtt/ml)
2. Calculate the flow rate in ml/hr.

DF = 15 gtt/ml
Ord = 2.5 μg/kg per min

Pertinent information provided: 2.5 μg/kg per min; 102 lb; 200 mg/250 ml

Unit equivalency conversion: 1000 μg/mg; 60 min/hr; 2.2 lb.kg; 15 gtt/ml
Desired units: (1)gtt/min; (2) ml/hr

CORRECT setup:

1. gtt/min:

$$\frac{15 \text{ gtt}}{\text{ml}} \times \frac{250 \text{ ml}}{200 \text{ mg}} \times \frac{\text{mg}}{1000 \text{ } \mu g} \times \frac{2.5 \text{ } \mu g}{\text{kg} \cdot \text{min}} \times \frac{\text{kg}}{2.2 \text{ lb}} \times 102 \text{ lb} = 2.2$$

$$= 2 \text{ gtt/min}$$

You cannot split a drop, so round the drip rates to the nearest drop.

Infusion pumps do not use decimals, so round the flow rates to the nearest whole number.

$DF \times A \times U \times Ord \times U \times BW = Ans$

2. ml/hr:

$$\frac{250 \text{ ml}}{200 \text{ mg}} \times \frac{\text{mg}}{1000 \text{ } \mu g} \times \frac{2.5 \text{ } \mu g}{\text{kg} \cdot \text{min}} \times \frac{60 \text{ min}}{\text{hr}} \times \frac{\text{kg}}{2.2 \text{ lb}} \times 102 \text{ lb} = 8.7 \text{ ml/hr}$$

$$= 9 \text{ ml/hr}$$

$A \times U \times Ord \times U \times U \times BW = Ans$

E X A M P L E   6

Dobutrex* HCl 10 μg/kg per min continuous IV infusion is ordered for your patient, who weighs 224 lb. Available is dobutamine HCl 250 mg in 250 ml of D$_5$W.

1. Calculate the number of gtt/min (10 gtt/ml).
2. Calculate the flow rate in ml/hr.

DF = 10 gtt/ml
Ord = 10 μg/kg per min

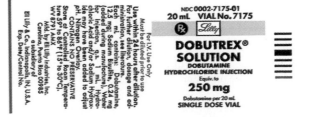

*Dobutrex® is a registered trademark of Eli Lilly and Company.

Pertinent information provided: 10 μg/kg per min; 224 lb; 250 mg/250 ml

Unit equivalency conversion: 1000 μg/mg; 2.2 lb/kg; 60 min/hr; 10 gtt/ml

Desired units: (1) ml/hr; (2) gtt/min

CORRECT setup:

1. gtt/min:

$$\frac{10 \text{ gtt}}{\text{ml}} \times \frac{250 \text{ ml}}{250 \text{ mg}} \times \frac{\text{mg}}{1000 \text{ } \mu g} \times \frac{10 \text{ } \mu g}{\text{kg} \cdot \text{min}} \times \frac{\text{kg}}{2.2 \text{ lb}} \times 224 \text{ lb} = 10.18$$

$$= 10 \text{ gtt/min}$$

DF × A × U ×
Ord × U ×
BW = Ans

2. ml/hr:

$$\frac{250 \text{ ml}}{250 \text{ mg}} \times \frac{\text{mg}}{1000 \text{ } \mu g} \times \frac{10 \text{ } \mu g}{\text{kg} \cdot \text{min}} \times \frac{60 \text{ min}}{\text{hr}} \times \frac{\text{kg}}{2.2 \text{ lb}} \times 224 \text{ lb} = 61.09$$

$$= 61 \text{ ml/hr}$$

A × U × Ord × U ×
U × BW = Ans

EXAMPLE 7

Quinidine 15 mg/kg over 4 hr is ordered as a loading dose, followed by 0.6 mg/kg per hr continuous IV infusion. Available is pharmacy-prepared quinidine 2 gm in 500 ml of D$_5$W. The patient weighs 174 lb.

Ord = 15 mg/kg
= 0.6 mg/kg per hr
Ov = 150 ml
Ot = 4 hr

1. Calculate the number of mg in the loading dose.
2. Calculate the flow rate in ml/hr for the loading dose.
3. Calculate the flow rate in ml/hr for the subsequent infusion.

Pertinent information provided: 15 mg/kg per 4hr; 0.6 mg/kg per hr; 174 lb; 2 gm/500 ml

Unit equivalency conversions: 1000 mg/gm; 2.2 lb/kg

Desired unit: ml/hr (loading and continuous infusion)

When in doubt, carry numbers to the second decimal place and round to the nearest measurable unit.

CORRECT setup:

1. mg/dose:

$$\frac{15 \text{ mg}}{\text{kg} \cdot \text{dose}} \times \frac{\text{kg}}{2.2 \text{ lb}} \times 174 \text{ lb} = 1186.36 \text{ mg/dose}$$

Ord × U × BW = Ans

2. ml/hr (loading):

$$\frac{500 \text{ ml}}{2 \text{ gm}} \times \frac{\text{gm}}{1000 \text{ mg}} \times \frac{15 \text{ mg}}{\text{kg} \cdot 4 \text{ hr}} \times \frac{\text{kg}}{2.2 \text{ lb}} \times 174 \text{ lb} = 74 \text{ ml/hr for 4 hr}$$

Ov × Ot = Ans

3. ml/hr (subsequent infusion):

$$\frac{500 \text{ ml}}{2 \text{ gm}} \times \frac{\text{gm}}{1000 \text{ mg}} \times \frac{0.6 \text{ mg}}{\text{kg} \cdot \text{hr}} \times \frac{\text{kg}}{2.2 \text{ lb}} \times 174 \text{ lb} = 11.9$$

$$= 12 \text{ ml/hr subsequent infusion}$$

A × U × Ord × U ×
BW = Ans

EXAMPLE 8

Diltiazem 15 mg/hr continuous IV infusion is ordered for your patient, who weighs 169 lb. Available is pharmacy-prepared diltiazem HCl 100 mg in 250 ml of D$_5$W. Calculate the number of gtt/min (15 gtt/ml) and the flow rate in ml/hr.

DF = 15 gtt/ml
Or = 15 mg/hr
A = 100 mg/250 ml

Pertinent information provided: 15 mg/hr; 100 mg/250 ml
Unit equivalency conversion: 60 min/hr; 15 gtt/ml
Desired units: (1) gtt/min; (2) ml/hr

CORRECT setup:

1. gtt/min:

$$\frac{15 \text{ gtt}}{\text{ml}} \times \frac{250 \text{ ml}}{100 \text{ mg}} \times \frac{15 \text{ mg}}{\text{hr}} \times \frac{\text{hr}}{60 \text{ min}} = 9.4 = 9 \text{ gtt/min}$$

2. ml/hr:

$$\frac{250 \text{ ml}}{100 \text{ mg}} \times \frac{15 \text{ mg}}{\text{hr}} = 37.5 = 38 \text{ ml/hr}$$

DF × A × Or × U =
Ans

A × Or = Ans

E X A M P L E   9

Isuprel 5 μg/min continuous IV infusion is ordered for your patient.
Available is isoproterenol HCl 1 mg in 500 ml of D$_5$W.

1. Calculate the number of gtt/min (15 gtt/ml).
2. Calculate the flow rate in ml/hr.

   Pertinent information provided: 5 μg/min; 1 mg/500 ml
   Unit equivalency conversion: 1000 μg/mg; 60 min/hr; 15 gtt/ml
   Desired units: (1) gtt/min; (2) ml/hr

Or = 5 μg/min
DF = 15 gtt/ml

CORRECT setup:

1. gtt/min:

$$\frac{15 \text{ gtt}}{\text{ml}} \times \frac{500 \text{ ml}}{1 \text{ mg}} \times \frac{\text{mg}}{1000 \text{ } \mu g} \times \frac{5 \text{ } \mu g}{\text{min}} = 37.5 = 38 \text{ gtt/min}$$

2. ml/hr:

$$\frac{500 \text{ ml}}{1 \text{ mg}} \times \frac{\text{mg}}{1000 \text{ } \mu g} \times \frac{5 \text{ } \mu g}{\text{min}} \times \frac{60 \text{ min}}{\text{hr}} = 150 \text{ ml/hr}$$

DF × A × U × Or =
Ans

A × U × Or × U = Ans

E X A M P L E   1 0

Abbokinase 4000 IU/min in 500 ml of NS for a 4-hr loading dose, then
1000 IU/min for 24 hr is ordered to treat arterial thrombosis. Available is
Abbokinase (urokinase) in vials of 250,000 IU and 500-ml unit bags of NS.

1. Calculate the number of IU needed for the entire order.
2. Calculate the flow rate of the loading dose in ml/hr.
3. Calculate the flow rate of subsequent doses in ml/hr.

   Pertinent information provided: 4000 IU/min; 1000 IU/min; 4 hr; 24 hr;
      500 ml; 250,000 IU/vial
   Unit equivalency conversion: 60 min/hr
   Desired units: (1) total mg of Abbokinase; (2) ml/hr loading dose;
      (3) ml/hr subsequent infusion

Or = 4000 IU/min load-
ing
Or = 4 hr loading
Ot = 24-hr continuous
infusion
Ov = 500 ml
A = Total calculated
dosage/Ov

CORRECT setup:

1. Total mg Abbokinase:

$$\frac{4000 \text{ IU}}{\text{min}} \times \frac{60 \text{ min}}{\text{hr}} \times 4 \text{ hr} = 960,000 \text{ IU in loading dose}$$

 Or × U × Ot = Ans (partial)

$$\frac{1000 \text{ IU}}{\text{min}} \times \frac{60 \text{ min}}{\text{hr}} \times 24 \text{ hr} = 1,440,000 \text{ IU for 24-hr infusion}$$

Total mg Abbokinase = 960,000 + 1,440,000 = 2,400,000 IU

 Or × U × Ot = Ans (partial)

2. ml/hr loading dose:

$$\frac{500 \text{ ml}}{2,400,000 \text{ IU}} \times \frac{4000 \text{ IU}}{\text{min}} \times \frac{60 \text{ min}}{\text{hr}} = 50 \text{ ml/hr loading}$$

 The sum of the loading dose plus 24 hr = Ans

3. ml/hr subsequent infusion:

$$\frac{500 \text{ ml}}{2,400,000 \text{ IU}} \times \frac{1000 \text{ IU}}{\text{min}} \times \frac{60 \text{ min}}{\text{hr}} = 12.5 = 13 \text{ ml/hr for next 24 hr}$$

 A × Or × U = Ans

Chapter Summary

This chapter has provided additional examples of in situ parenteral dosage administration. The scenarios represent medications frequently ordered in hospitals (inpatient settings) and clinic settings (outpatient settings). The process of calculating dosages using dimensional analysis (DA) remains the same, whether the problem is asking you to calculate oral, injectable, or parenteral dosages.

You will need to keep these points in mind when you are solving these types of problems:

✔ Extract pertinent information.
✔ Rewrite the facts as conversion factors.
✔ Add the necessary unit equivalency conversion factors.
✔ Set up all the conversion factors in a continuous chain to allow unwanted units to cancel.

If you are still having problems in calculating dosages using DA, consider the following suggestions:

✔ Implement the process to cancel the unwanted units in the unit equivalency conversions, for example; lb to kg, kg to mg, mg to µg, min to hr, ml to L.

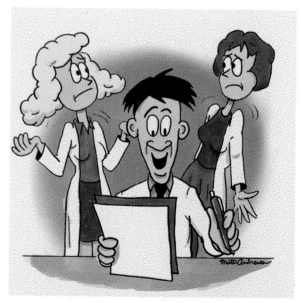

"LET'S SEE... 20% FOR FOOD, 40% FOR RENT, 20% FOR MY CAR PAYMENT, 20% FOR UTILITIES, AND 10% FOR SAVINGS.... WOW! THAT LEAVES ME 20% FOR SPENDING!"

✔ Shorten the chains in the conversion unit setups, by doing the unit equivalency conversions first and then using the converted units in your final setup.

✔ Do not give up! Review Chapters 2 through 5 again.

✔ Practice the DA process by using it in all your

other daily calculations; for example, if the price of gasoline is \$1.38/gal and you have \$10.00 to spend, calculate the number of gal of gas you can purchase:

$$\frac{gal}{\$1.38} \times \$10.00 = 7.2 \text{ gal}$$

PROBLEM SET	PROBLEM SET ANSWERS
1. Ordered: Lidocaine HCl 75 mg IV bolus Available: Xylocaine HCl 100 mg/5 ml Calculate the number of ml/dose.	1. 3.7 ml/dose
2. Ordered: Lidocaine 2 mg/min continuous IV infusion Available: Xylocaine 2 gm in 500 ml of D₅W a. Calculate the flow rate in ml/hr.	2. a. 30 ml/hr
b. Calculate the number of gtt/min (15 gtt/ml).	b. 7.5 = 8 gtt/min
3. Ordered: Garamycin 80 mg IVPB over 30 min t.i.d. Available Garamycin (gentamicin sulfate) 80 mg in 50 ml of D₅W a. Calculate the flow rate in ml/hr.	3. a. 100 ml/hr
b. Calculate the number of gtt/min (15 gtt/ml).	b. 25 gtt/min

PROBLEM SET	PROBLEM SET ANSWERS

4. Ordered: Heparin 5000 U IV at 1200 U/hr
    Available: Heparin 5000 U in 500 ml of D_5W
    a. Calculate the number of ml/hr.

    b. Calculate the number of gtt/min (10 gtt/ml).

5. Ordered: DTIC-Dome 2 mg/kg IVPB over 30 min q.d. for 10 d for your patient, who weighs 103 lb
    Available: Dacarbazine 10 mg/ml reconstituted in 100 ml of NS
    Calculate the number of ml of DTIC-Dome/dose.

6. Ordered: Mustargen 400 μg/kg IVSP single dose for your patient, who weighs 132 lb
    Available: Mechlorethamine HCl 1 mg/ml reconstituted
    Calculate the number of ml/dose.

7. Ordered: Blenoxane 0.25 U/kg IVSP over 10 min for your patient, who weighs 115 lb
    Available: Bleomycin sulfate 15 U/5ml reconstituted with NS
    Calculate the number of ml/dose.

Answers:

4. a. 120 ml/hr
    b. 20 gtt/min

5. Add 9.4 ml of DTIC-Dome into 100 ml of NS.

6. 2.4 ml/dose

7. 4.4 ml/dose

PROBLEM SET	PROBLEM SET ANSWERS
8. Ordered: Cerubidine 45 mg/m² per d IVSP through a port on a free-flowing primary IV system, for a patient who weighs 141 lb and measures 5′2″ Available: Daunorubicin HCl 5 mg/ml reconstituted a. What is the patient's BSA?	8. a. 1.72 m²
b. Calculate the number of mg/dose.	b. 77.4 mg/dose
c. Calculate the number of ml/dose.	c. 15.5 ml/dose
9. Ordered: Mutamycin 20 mg/m² per dose IVSP over 5 min, repeat every 6 wk, for a patient whose BSA is 1.58 m² Available: Mutamycin 0.5 mg/ml reconstituted vials, already diluted to 20 μg/ml according to instruction a. Calculate the number of mg/dose.	9. a. 31.6 mg/dose b. 63 ml/dose
b. Calculate the number of ml/dose.	

PROBLEM SET

10. Ordered: Mithracin 25 $\mu g/kg$ in 1 L of D_5W over 6 hr for your patient, who weighs 172 lb
Available: Mithracin (plicamycin) 2.5 mg/5 ml reconstituted
a. Calculate the number of ml Mithracin/dose.

b. Calculate the flow rate in ml/hr.

11. Ordered: Cytosar-U 100 mg/m^2 per d continuous IV infusion for 5 d, for a patient whose BSA is 1.86 m^2
Available: Cytarabine 1 gm/20 ml reconstituted, diluted with 1 L of NS
a. Calculate the total number of mg for the 5-day dose.

b. Calculate the flow rate in ml/hr.

c. Calculate the drip rate in μgtt/min.

PROBLEM SET ANSWERS

10. a. 3.9 ml/dose
b. 166.7 = 167 ml/hr

11. a. 930 mg
b. 8.5 ml/hr
c. 8.5 = 9 μgtt/min

PROBLEM SET	PROBLEM SET ANSWERS
12. Ordered: Procainamide HCl 20 mg/min, max total 17 mg/kg continuous IV infusion, for a patient who weighs 159 lb Available: Procan 2 gm/4 ml, and D₅W 500-ml unit bag a. Calculate the number of ml of procainamide HCl to add to the 500 ml of D₅W.	12. a. Add 2.5 ml procain-amide HCl to the 500 ml of D₅W. b. 1.2 gm of procain-amide HCl c. 489 ml/hr
b. Convert ml of procainamide HCl to the equivalent gm of procain-amide HCl.	
c. Calculate the flow rate in ml/hr.	
13. Ordered: Sodium bicarbonate 1 mEq/kg IVSP over 60 min, for a patient who weighs 187 lb Available: 1 mEq/ml in 50-ml vials a. Calculate the number of ml/dose.	13. a. 85 ml/dose b. 1.4 ml/min
b. Calculate the number of ml/min.	

PROBLEM SET

14. Ordered: Lidocaine 1.5 mg/kg (max 100 mg/dose) IV bolus, repeat q3–5 min (total loading dose of 3 mg/kg), for a patient who weighs 178 lb
    Available: Lidocaine 100 mg/5 ml
    Calculate the dosage in ml/dose.

14. 121 mg > 100 mg/dose: the patient will receive the maximum dose of 100 mg/dose. The number of ml/dose = 5 ml.

15. Ordered: Quinidine gluconate 15 mg/kg in D_5W over 6 hr, for a patient who weighs 135 lb
    Available: Quinaglute 2 gm in 500 ml of D_5W
    a. Calculate the number of mg/dose.

15. a. 920 mg/dose
    b. You will need to administer only 230 ml of the available 500 ml.
    c. 38 ml/hr
    d. 9.6 = 10 gtt/min

    b. Calculate the number of ml/dose from 2 gm/500 ml.

    c. Calculate the flow rate in ml/hr.

    d. Calculate the number of gtt/min (15 gtt/ml).

PROBLEM SET	PROBLEM SET ANSWERS

16. Ordered: Nipride 5 μg/kg per min continuous IV infusion, for a patient who weighs 215 lb
Available: Nitroprusside sodium 500 mg in 250 ml of D_5W
a. Calculate the number of mg/hr.
 	
b. Calculate the number of ml/hr.
 	
c. Calculate the number of μgtt/min (60 μgtt/ml).
	16. a. 29.3 = 29 mg/hr
	     b. 15 ml/hr
	     c. 15 μgtt/min

17. Ordered: Tridil 5 μg/min continuous IV infusion Available: Nitroglycerin 5 mg in 500 ml of D_5W a. Calculate the number of μgtt/min. b. Calculate the flow rate in ml/hr.	17. a. 30 μgtt/min b. 30 ml/hr

PROBLEM SET	PROBLEM SET ANSWERS

18. Ordered: Furosemide 1 mg/kg IVSP bolus, for a patient who weighs 178 lb
Available: Lasix 1 gm in 250 ml of NS
a. Calculate the number of mg/bolus dose.

18. a. 80.9 = 81 mg/bolus dose
b. 20.25 = 20 ml/bolus dose

b. Calculate the number of ml/bolus dose.

19. Ordered: Wellcovorin 20 mg/m^2 IV q6hr for 21 d for a patient whose BSA is 1.57 m^2
Available: Leucovorin calcium 100 mg/ml
a. Calculate the number of mg/dose.

19. a. 31.4 mg/dose
b. 2637.5 mg = 2.6 gm for the entire 21 d

b. Calculate the number of gm for the entire 21-day order.

20. Ordered: Pentam 4 mg/kg (max 300 mg) in 100 ml over 1 hr q.d. for 21 d, for a patient who weighs 107 lb
Available: 300-mg vials of Pentam (pentamidine isethionate)
a. Calculate the number of mg/dose.

20. a. 194.5 = 195 gm/dose
b. 25 gtt/min

b. Calculate the drip rate in gtt/min (15 gtt/ml).

PROBLEM SET	PROBLEM SET ANSWERS

21. Ordered: Pavulon 0.3 mg/kg per hr continuous IV infusion for a patient who weighs 154 lb
    Available: Pancuronium bromide 50 mg in 100 ml of D_5W
    a. Calculate the number of mg/hr.

    b. Calculate the number of ml/hr.

    c. How many hr and min will the available dosage last for this order?

21. a. 21 mg/hr
    b. 42 ml/hr
    c. 2 hr and 23 min

22. Ordered: Magnesium sulfate 2 gm IVSP at 150 mg/min
    Available: Magnesium sulfate of 20% solution
    a. Calculate the number of ml/min.

    b. Calculate the total time necessary to administer the order.

22. a. 0.75 = 0.8 ml/min
    b. 13.33 min to administer the order

PROBLEM SET	PROBLEM SET ANSWERS

23. Ordered: Phenobarbital sodium 15 mg/kg over 20 min for a patient who weighs 145 lb
Available: Phenobarbital sodium in reconstituted vials of 120 mg/3 ml
a. Calculate the number of mg/dose.

23. a. 988 mg/dose
b. 2.7 = 3 vials of phenobarbital sodium
c. 8.2 ml/dose. You will only need 0.2 ml from the third vial.
d. 74.1 = 74 ml/hr

b. Calculate the number of vials necessary for this order.

c. Calculate the number of reconstituted phenobarbital sodium ml/dose.

d. Calculate the number of ml/hr.

24. Ordered: Nitroprusside sodium 0.6 μg/kg per min continuous IV infusion, for a patient who weighs 138 lb
Available: Nitroprusside sodium 50 mg/250 ml of D_5W
a. Calculate the flow rate in ml/hr.

24. a. 11.29 = 11 ml/hr
b. 11.29 = 11 μgtt/min

b. Calculate the drip rate in μgtt/min.

PROBLEM SET	PROBLEM SET ANSWERS

25. Ordered: Kytril 1 mg in 50 ml of D_5W over 20 min
     Available: Single-dose vials of Kytril (granisetron HCl) 1 mg/ml
     a. Calculate the drip rate in gtt/min (15 gtt/ml).

     b. Calculate the drip rate in gtt/sec.

     c. Calculate the drip rate in whole gtt/time in sec.

25. a. 37.5 = 38 gtt/min
     b. 0.625 gtt/sec
     c. 5 gtt/8 sec

26. Ordered: Insulin 8 U/hr continuous IV infusion
     Available: Humulin R 200 U in 500 ml of NS
     a. Calculate the flow rate in ml/hr.

     b. Calculate the number of μgtt/min.

     c. Calculate the number of whole μgtt/time in sec.

26. a. 20 ml/hr
     b. 20 μgtt/min
     c. 20 μgtt/60 sec = 1 μgtt/3 sec

PROBLEM SET	PROBLEM SET ANSWERS

27. Ordered: NS 100 ml/hr continuous IV infusion
Available: NS 1-L unit bag
a. Calculate the number of hr of infusion of NS per 1-L unit bag.

b. The infusion was started at 7:30 AM, so when will you need to administer the next unit bag?

28. Ordered: D$_5$ ½ NS via a 1-L bolus (over 1 hr)
Available: D$_5$ ½ NS in a 1-L unit bag.
a. Calculate the number of gtt/min (15 gtt/ml).

b. Calculate the number of gtt/sec.

29. Ordered: D$_5$ ½ NS 1 L over 24 hr (NS = 0.9% = 154 mEq of sodium/L)
Available: D$_5$W in a 1-L unit bag
    NaCl 4 mEq/ml in a 50-ml vial
Calculate the number of ml of NaCl 4 mEq that you will need to make the IV solution for this order.

PROBLEM SET ANSWERS

27. a. 10 hr
    b. 5:30 PM

28. a. 250 gtt/min
    b. 4.16 = 4 gtt/sec (close to impossible to count clean drops)

29. Add 19.25 = 19.3 ml of NaCl 4 mEq to the 1-L unit bag of D$_5$W.

PROBLEM SET	PROBLEM SET ANSWERS

30. Ordered: D_5 ¼ NS with 20 mEq of KCl continuous infusion at 120 ml/hr
Available: D_5W in a 1-L unit bag; NaCl 4 mEq/ml in a 50-ml vial; KCl 40 mEq in a 20-ml vial
a. Calculate the number of ml of NaCl 4 mEq/L D_5W.

30. a. Add 9.6 ml of NaCl 4 mEq/ml to 1 L of D_5W, and then
b. Add 10 ml of KCl stock to the same 1 L of D_5W.

b. Calculate the number of ml of KCl 40 mEq/20 ml.

Scenarios in Critical and Intensive Care Medication Dosages

31. a. A man who weighs 66 kg is prescribed a 2 mg/min drip of lidocaine for ventricular bigeminy. The concentration available is 1000 mg/250 cc D_5W. How many cc/hr of lidocaine do you administer?

31. a. 30 cc/hr
b. 22.5 = 23 cc/hr

b. The patient rapidly progresses to intermittent ventricular tachycardia despite boluses, and 4 mg/min drip of lidocaine. The physician now prescribes a bolus of 1000 mg of procainamide followed by a 3 mg/min IV drip. The available concentration is 2000 mg/250 cc of D_5W. How many cc/hr of procainamide do you administer?

PROBLEM SET	PROBLEM SET ANSWERS

32. a. A patient who weighs 55 kg and has undergone CABG (coronary artery bypass graft) × 4 has an order for dobutamine to be titrated to keep her cardiac index above 2.0. Currently, the available concentration and IV drip rate is 500 mg/250 cc of D_5W running at 8 cc/hr. How many µg/kg per min is the patient receiving.

32. a. 4.8 µg/kg per min
     b. 4.95 = 5 cc/hr

   b. The physician orders you to titrate down and maintain the dobutamine drip at 3 µg/kg per min. How many cc/hr is this?

33. a. A teenager who weighs 72 kg is in septic shock. His current blood pressure (BP) is 75/40. A dopamine drip (800 mg/500 cc of D_5W) is prescribed for 5 µg/kg per min by the physician. How many ml/hr do you administer?

33. a. 13.50 = 14 ml/hr
     b. 11 µg/kg per min

   b. The physician at the bedside observes no response from the dopamine drip. He states "Increase his dopamine drip to 15 cc/hr." How many µg/kg per min is the patient now receiving?

PROBLEM SET	PROBLEM SET ANSWERS

34. a. The physician orders a heparin infusion of 30,000 U per day for a patient diagnosed with a pulmonary embolism. The pharmacy delivers 1000 cc of NS. How many U/hr of heparin should this patient receive?

34. a. 1250 U/hr
b. 42 cc/hr

b. How many cc/hr of heparin do you administer?

35. a. Sodium nitroprusside 800 mg/250 ml of D_5W is ordered for a 68-kg woman with a BP of 170/88 who has emerged from anesthesia after mitral valve replacement (MVR) and coronary venous graft (CVG) × 2. The initial order reads "Nipride, 3 μg/kg per min initially titrated to keep systolic BP between 100 and 110." Initially, how many cc/hr should you administer?

35. a. 3.8 = 4 cc/hr
b. 7 μg/kg per min

b. You have titrated the sodium nitroprusside to 9 cc/hr to maintain your patient's therapeutic blood pressure. How many μg/kg per min is this?

Some Facts About Medication Calculation Using DA

1. The five rights and the three checks, along with the nursing process, must be applied to the administration of medications.
2. Apply the nursing process as it relates to administering medications.
3. Most chemotherapeutic agents are toxic to the cell, that is, cytotoxic.
4. Institutional safety standards and protocols on toxic chemicals are designed to protect both human life and the environment.
5. Chemotherapeutic agents must be handled within the guidelines of hazardous chemicals and safety protocols and discarded into toxic/hazardous waste receptacles.
6. If you discover an infiltrate at the IV site, stop the IV. If the medication is cytotoxic, the site many need to be detoxified.
7. Gastric lavage via orogastric tube, with or without activated charcoal, is administered to prevent diffuse absorption of poisons.
8. Syrup of ipecac induces vomiting.
9. Chelation therapy with a chelating agent removes heavy metals and other highly ionized molecules from the circulatory system, that is, heavy metal poisoning induced by elements such as lead or mercury.
10. The advanced cardiac life-support (ACLS) algorithm provides guidelines for the administration of basic life-support measures, namely, electro- and chemical cardioversion and endotracheal intubation.
11. Medications used during ACLS for chemical cardioversion and/or resuscitation require constant monitoring of the patient's cardiac and/or circulatory response.
12. Medication dosage orders for cardiac and circulatory resuscitations can change rapidly, depending on the patient's response.
13. The abbreviation for endotracheal administration is ET; intraperitoneal administration is IP; intrathecal (intraspinal) administration is IT.
14. Oral medication can be administered through a nasogastric tube to patients who are unable to ingest the medication.
15. The sizes of orogastric and nasogastric tubes are positively correlated with the accompanying unit measurement of the French tube, that is, the larger the number, the larger the lumen.
16. Place the desired unit first and in proper orientation in your setup.
17. Always double-check your math. Take the time to recalculate; it may make the difference between a correct and an incorrect dose.

5. The provider has ordered an increase in the dosage of Hytrin (terazosin HCl) from 2 mg to 4 mg q.h.s. for Mr. Nash. He still has 36 of the Hytrin 2-mg tab. How many days' supply of pills does he have?

6. K-Dur (potassium chloride) 20 mg PO q.d. is ordered for Mrs. O'Neil. Her caregiver wants to know if she can crush the tab and mix it with some applesauce. You know that K-Dur has a controlled-release system. What will you tell her?

7. Mr. Duvall is receiving Pepto-Bismol (bismuth subsalicylate) PO as part of a treatment regimen for a duodenal ulcer caused by *Helicobacter pylori.* You have instructed him to take 525 mg PO q.i.d., 1 hr before meals and at bedtime. The medication comes in a 262-mg tab.

   a. How many tab should Mr. Duvall take in 24 hr?

   b. The treatment regimen is to continue for 14 days. The medication can be purchased over the counter and in a package of 30 tab.
   How many packages will this patient need to purchase for 14 d of medication?

8. Pravachol (pravastatin sodium) 20 mg q.h.s. is ordered for Mrs. Weinstein's hyperlipidemia. The pharmacist has called to ask if Pravachol 10-mg tab can be given instead of 20-mg tab. How many tab will Mrs. Weinstein need to take each night?

9. Mrs. Jensen is to have 5 gtt of V̄oSol Otic (acetic acid) solution 2% instilled in her left ear q.i.d. The pharmacy sends you a 5-ml bottle of V̄oSol Otic 2% solution. Calculate the total number of doses from the volume in the bottle (15 gtt/ml).

10. Morphine sulfate gr $^1/_{15}$ is ordered. Morphine sulfate comes in ampules of 6 mg/ml. Calculate the number of ml/dose.

11. Acetazolamide is a diuretic, antiglaucoma, and anticonvulsant agent. The order reads: Diamox 250 mg PO t.i.d. The pharmacy sends you Diamox SR 500-mg capsules (cap). What will you do?

12. Albuterol 0.5 ml in 2.5 ml of NS for oral inhalation via a nebulizer q.i.d. p.r.n. is ordered for an acute exacerbation of asthma. Available is Proventil 0.5% solution. Calculate the number of mg/dose.

13. Mr. Lee was taking Paxil (paroxetine HCl) 20 mg/day in the morning for his depression. A week later, the provider ordered a dosage increase of 10 mg/d. Paxil is available in 10-mg tab. Calculate the number of tab/dose.

14. Mr. Torres walks into the ER complaining of an itchy rash all over his body. You take one look at the rash and suspect chickenpox. Quickly, you usher him into an examination room, taking care to minimize his exposure to other patients. The nurse practitioner orders Zovirax 800 mg PO 5 times a day for 1 wk. How many gm of acyclovir will Mr. Torres have taken by the end of a week?

15. While in the hospital, Mrs. Sanchez received Mylanta (aluminum hydroxide; magnesium hydroxide; simethicone) 30 ml PO p.r.n. for relief of heartburn. She has told you that she takes 3 teaspoons (tsp) of Mylanta at home for relief, and she wants to know if she is taking enough. Please figure it out, so you can instruct her accurately.

16. For the prevention of osteoporosis, Mrs. Schneider is taking Premarin (conjugated estrogens) 0.625 mg PO q.d. on a cycle of 3-weeks-on, and 1-week-off. How many gm of estrogen will she receive by the end of the fourth week?

17. Synthroid 0.3 mg PO q.d. is ordered for Mrs. Rodriguez for treatment of hypothyroidism. The pharmacist calls to tell you that the pharmacy is out of Synthroid 0.3 mg. Available is levothyroxine sodium 0.1 mg. How many tab does Mrs. Rodriguez have to take each day until the proper dosage is available?

18. For Mrs. Sighn's gastric ulcer, the doctor ordered Prilosec (omeprazole) 20 mg PO b.i.d. The pharmacist filled the prescription with Prilosec 10-mg capsules (cap). Calculate the number of cap/d.

19. The doctor ordered digoxin 0.15 mg intravenous slow push (IVSP) stat. You have in stock digoxin 500 μg/2 ml. Calculate the number of ml/dose.

20. Zantac (ranitidine HCl) 150 mg PO b.i.d. is ordered for Mr. Noonan's duodenal ulcer. Available is Zantac 75 mg/5 ml syrup. Calculate the number of tsp/dose.

21. For Mr. Hansen's prostate infection, the provider ordered Cipro (ciprofloxacin) 500 mg PO b.i.d. for 2 wk. Available is Cipro 500-mg tab. How many tab will Mr. Hansen need to take in order to complete this course of antibiotic treatment?

22. Furosemide 160 mg intravenous slow push (IVSP) was ordered for an exacerbation of Mrs. Smith's congestive heart failure (CHF). Available is furosemide in vials of 100 mg/10 ml.

    a. How many ml will you need to draw for this order?

    b. How many vials will you need for this order?

23. Voltaren (diclofenac sodium) is a nonsteroidal anti-inflammatory agent. The order is for Voltaren 50 mg PO t.i.d. for the control of joint pain. The patient was given 25-mg tab of Voltaren. How many tab will the patient need for each dose?

24. Milrinone 50 μg/kg IVSP over 10 min was ordered for Mrs. Pugh, who weighs 286 lb. Available is Primacor 1 mg/ml. How many ml will you need to give Mrs. Pugh?

25. It is your turn to make the cooling alcohol sponge-bath solution. The pharmacy sends you a pint of their stock solution of 95% ethanol (ETOH). After having the delivery form countersigned, you start to dilute the stock solution to make 1 pint of 10% ETOH solution (1 pt = 480 ml).

    a. How many ml of stock ETOH will you need to make 1 pint of this solution?

    b. Calculate the number of ml of water to add.

    c. Calculate the number of pt of 10% ETOH you can make from 1 pt of stock 95% ETOH.

26. Mrs. Jones is to receive 45 mg of an IM medication. It is available only in vials of 75 mg/2 ml. How many ml need to be administered?

27. Morphine 8 mg IM q4hr is the order. You have in stock morphine 15 mg/ml. Calculate the number of ml/dose.

28. An insulin order reads 30 units of NPH Insulin SQ stat. The label on the Humulin NPH vial reads 1 ml = 100 units. What will be an appropriate size of insulin syringe for this order?

29. Sus-Phrine (epinephrine) 1:200, 0.15 ml SQ stat is ordered for the treatment of anaphylaxis. Available is Sus-Phrine 1:200. Calculate the number of ml/dose.

30. The order for the loading dose reads aminophhylline 5.6 mg/kg of total body weight in 100 ml of D₅W IV over 20-min infusion time. Your patient weighs 105 lb. Calculate the number of mg of aminophylline needed for this patient.

31. In the treatment of AIDS-related Kaposi's sarcoma, the recommended induction dose of Roferon-A (interferon alpha 2-A) is 36 million IU IM q.d. You are out of the vials of 36 million/ml. Instead, you have in stock 10 vials of 9 million IU/ml. How many vials do you need for this order?

32. In the treatment of hairy cell leukemia, the induction dose of Roferon-A is 3 million IU SQ daily for 16 to 24 weeks. Roferon-A is available in a dosage of 18 million IU per vial reconstituted to a total of 3 ml. Calculate the number of ml/dose.

33. The recommended premedication dose of Versed (midazolam HCl) is 0.07 mg/kg IM 1 hr before surgery. Available is Versed 50 mg/10 ml. Mrs. Klosky weighs 149 lb. Calculate the number of ml/dose.

34. Terramycin (oxytetracycline HCl) 250 mg IM q.d. is ordered for Mr. Miranda. Available is Terramycin for injection in glass ampules of 250 mg/2 ml. Calculate the number of cc/dose.

35. You are taking inventory of the stock medication cupboard and you come across a bottle of glucose solution labeled 1:5. Calculate the concentration in mg/ml.

36. You are making an NS solution for an NS wet-to-dry dressing change. You have sterilized the water (by boiling) and you have available a pharmaceutical grade of sodium chloride (NaCl) crystals. You know that NS is a 0.9% solution. Calculate the number of mg of NaCl for 1 L of NS.

37. Nitroprusside sodium 0.6 μg/kg per min is ordered for Mrs. Salud, who weighs 128 lb. Available is nitroprusside sodium 50 mg/250 ml of NS. Calculate the number of μgtt/min.

38. Kytril (granisetron HCl) 1 mg in 50 cc of D₅W over 15 min was ordered for Mrs. Wynn. Calculate the drip rate in μgtt/min (15 gtt/ml).

39. Calcium gluconate comes in a vial of 1 gm/10 ml. The order is to give 320 mg of calcium gluconate IVSP. Calculate the number of ml/dose.

40. Zofran (ondansetron HCl) 20 mg in 50 ml of D₅W over 15 min for the prevention of nausea was ordered prior to chemotherapy. Calculate the drip rate in gtt/min (10 gtt/ml).

41. D₅W 80 ml/hr is ordered for Mrs. Scott. How many kcal will she receive from the dextrose in a day if each gm of dextrose provides 3.75 kcal?

42. An insulin drip of 8 units/hr is ordered for Mr. Moore. Available is Humulin R 200 U/500 ml of NS. Calculate the flow rate in ml/hr for this patient.

43. Alprostadil 0.1 µg/kg per min continuous IV infusion is ordered for little Bobby for the temporary maintenance of a patent ductus arteriosus while the infant is awaiting surgery. Available is alprostadil 500 µg/250 ml of NS. Little Bobby weighs 5 lb 6 oz.

   a. Convert little Bobby's body weight to kg.

   b. Calculate the drip rate in µgtt/min.

44. The maintenance dose of aminophylline is 5 mg/kg per day IV q12hr administered via a small-volume administration system. Available is aminophylline 50 mg/50 ml of D₅W. Tiny Joey weighs 4 lb 13 oz.

   a. Convert Joey's body weight to kg.

   b. Calculate the number of ml/dose.

45. The patient's ECG reveals a change from arrhythmia to torsades de pointes. The emergency room (ER) doctor initiates the cardioversion process by asking for magnesium sulfate 2 gm IV bolus over 5 min. Available is magnesium sulfate 50% solution in 10-ml vials. Calculate the number of ml/dose for loading.

46. NS 100 ml/hr continuous IV infusion is ordered and started at 1:00 PM with a 1-L unit bag of NS. How long will it be before you need to hang the next bag?

47. Lidocaine 75 mg IV bolus is ordered for an arrhythmia. The patient weighs 50 kg. Available is Xylocaine in vials of 100 mg/5 ml. Calculate the number of ml/bolus dose.

48. For maintenance, lidocaine 2 mg/min continuous IV infusion is ordered. Available is Xylocaine 2 gm/500 ml of D_5W. Calculate the number of gtt/min (15 gtt/ml).

49. Decadron 10 mg/50 ml of D_5W over 20 min is ordered for Mrs. Kline. Decadron comes in vials of 24 mg/ml and unit bags of D_5W 50 ml.

    a. Calculate the number of ml of Decadron for this order.

    b. Calculate the drip rate in gtt/min (15 gtt/ml).

50. Heparin 5000 units at 1200 U/hr is ordered. Available is heparin 5000 U/100 ml D_5W. Calculate the flow rate in ml/hr.

51. Garamycin 80 mg IVPB over 60 min t.i.d. is ordered. Available is Garamycin 80 mg in 100 ml of D_5W. Calculate the drip rate in gtt/min (15 gtt/ml).

52. A solution of D_5W in ¼ NS with 20 mEq KCl 1 L/d is ordered. You have available D_5W in 250-cc unit bags; NaCl in vials of 4 mEq/ml and KCl in vials of 40 mEq/20 ml. Normal saline 0.9% has NaCl 154 mEq/L.

    a. Calculate the number of ml of NaCl you will need to add to the 250 ml of D_5W.

    b. Calculate the number of ml of KCl you will need to add to the IV solution.

    c. Calculate the flow rate in ml/hr.

53. The order is for a D_5W bolus at 500 ml/hr for 4 hr followed by KVO at 500 ml/12 hr. Available is D_5W in a 1-L unit bag.

    a. Calculate the drip rates in gtt/min for the bolus dose.

    b. Calculate the drip rates to KVO (15 gtt/ml).

54. Jamie, a 16-year-old math whiz, counted the drops of IV fluid entering the drip chamber from the bag. She counted 20 drops each minute and asked you how much that is in fl oz/d (15 gtt/ml).

55. A solution of D_5W in ½ NS with 20mEq of KCl in 1 L at 100 ml/hr is ordered. Available are D_5W 500-ml unit bags; NaCl 4 mEq/ml; and KCl 2 mEq/ml. (NS = 154 mEq of NaCl/L.)

a. Calculate the number of ml of NaCl to add to the 500-ml unit bag of D_5W.

b. Calculate the number of ml of KCl to add to the 500-ml unit bag of D_5W.

56. Heather received a new 500-ml bag of D_5W at 9:00 PM. The order is to give 500 ml/8 hr. Calculate the flow rate in ml/hr.

57. Aminophylline loading dose is 6 mg/kg total body weight in 100 ml of D_5W IVPB over 20 min. Tim, an 11-year-old boy, weighs 75 lb. Available is aminophylline in vials of 250 mg/10 ml.

a. Calculate the number of ml in the aminophylline loading dose.

b. Calculate the number of gtt/min (15 gtt/ml).

58. Two gm of magnesium sulfate in 50 ml of D_5W over 20 min was ordered. Calculate the drip rate gtt/min (10 gtt/ml).

59. At 7:00 AM, Mrs. Austin began receiving 1 L of D_5W at 100 ml/hr. At 10:00 AM, Rocephin 1 gm/50 ml IVPB over 30 min was administered. Calculate the total amount of IV fluid received between 7:00 and 10:30 AM.

60. The night-shift nurse was running late, and stated that no entry of fluid intake for Mrs. Austin had been made since 4:00 PM the previous day (see Q. 59). The night-shift nurse has asked that you do her a big favor by completing the fluid intake sheet. On the run, she has told you that the change in order from D_5W 100 ml/hr to D_5W in NS 2 L/d took place at 11:00 PM. What will be your entry for Mrs. Austin's fluid intake between the 4:00 PM yesterday and 7:00 AM today?

61. An infusion of hydrocortisone 5 mg/kg in 50 ml of NS IV q8hr over 30 min is ordered for a nonanaphylactic, severe allergic response. Mr. Lum weighs 136 lb. Available is Hydrocortone Phosphate 50 mg/ml. Calculate the number of ml of Hydrocortone Phosphate to add to the 50-ml unit bag of NS.

62. The order is for IV Rocephin (ceftriaxone sodium) to be administered over 30 min. Available are Rocephin 500-mg vials. The direction for reconstitution calls for 4.8 ml of IV solution to yield 5 ml of Rocephin. Calculate the number of mg/ml in the reconstituted Rocephin.

63. Rocephin 2 gm in 50 ml IVPB over 30 min is ordered. Available is Rocephin in a 1-gm vial reconstituted to 10 ml.

   a. Calculate the number of vial/dose.

   b. Calculate the number of gtt/min (15 gtt/ml)

64. Valium (diazepam) 5 mg IVSP over 1 min is ordered. Valium comes in ampules of 10 mg/2 ml. Calculate the number of ml/dose.

65. Cefobid 2 gm in NS at a concentration of 20 mg/ml IVPB b.i.d. over 30 min is ordered. Available is a 2-gm vial of Cefobid sterile powder that requires 2.8 ml/gm diluent.

   a. Calculate the number of ml of diluent for the available Cefobid dosage form.

   b. Calculate the number of ml of NS needed to further dilute 2 gm of Cefobid for administration.

   c. Calculate the flow rate in ml/hr.

66. Emete-con (benzoquinamide HCl) is ordered to treat the nausea and vomiting associated with anesthesia and surgery. The dosage is 0.2 mg/kg IVSP over 1 min. Emete-con is available in a 10-mg vial. The direction for reconstitution is 2.2 ml of sterile water to yield 2 ml of solution. Your patient, Mr. Moon, weighs 220 lb. How many ml of Emete-con will he receive?

67. Cefuroxime 1.5 gm IVPB over 30 min is ordered for treating Mrs. Smith's periorbital cellulitis. Mrs. Smith weighs 128 lb. Cefuroxime was delivered to you in the concentration of 1.5 gm/100 ml of NS. Calculate the drip rate in gtt/min for this infusion (15 gtt/ml).

68. Mr. Noyce is to receive an insulin drip at a rate of 4 units/hr. Available is 200 units of Regular Insulin in 250 ml of NS. Calculate the insulin flow rate in ml/hr.

69. You came onto the short-stay unit at the beginning of your shift at 6:00 AM and found Mrs. Winston being infused with a bag of lactated Ringer's solution (LR) with a macrodrip set at 2 gtt/sec (15 gtt/ml). You estimated the amount of LR solution left to infuse at 450 ml. When will you hang a new bag of LR solution?

70. It is 2:00 PM. Mr. Brown, who is in a short-stay unit, is to receive 1 L of NS continuous IV infusion at 250 ml/hr, and then is to be discharged. The drop factor is 15 gtt/ml. She wants to know when her IV needle will be removed. How many hours and minutes will it take to infuse this bag of IV solution?

71. Dobutamine hydrochloride 500 mg in 250 ml of D_5W continuous IV at 10 μg/kg per min is ordered for Mrs. Oldes, who weighs 97 lb. Calculate the flow rate in ml/hr.

72. Esmolol 100 μg/kg per min IV infusion was ordered for Mrs. Torres, who weighs 190 lb. Available is esmolol 2.5 gm in 500 ml of D_5NS.

    a. Calculate the drip rate in gtt/min (15 gtt/ml).

    b. Calculate the flow rate in ml/hr.

73. Mr. Lee is to receive IV heparin. The physician ordered 20,000 units of heparin in 500 ml of D_5W to be infused at the rate of 1000 units/hr. Calculate the flow rate in ml/hr.

74. Adriamycin (doxorubicin HCl) 20 mg/m^2 is ordered for Mrs. Cortez, who is 5'3" tall and weighs 142 lb. You are double-checking what the pharmacy sent you, Adriamycin 34 mg in 50 cc of D_5W. The nomogram figures Mrs. Cortez's body surface area (BSA) to be 1.7 m^2. Did you receive the correct dosage from the pharmacy?

75. Little Jose weighs 66 lb. Epinephrine (1:10,000) 0.01 mg/kg IV q5min is ordered to treat his sinus bradycardia. Calculate the number of mg of epinephrine/dose.

76. Cody, who is 3 years old, has an elevated temperature. The standing order/protocol for children's Tylenol (acetaminophen) is 1 gr/year of age PO q.i.d. Available is children's Tylenol elixir 120 mg/5 ml. Calculate the number of tsp/dose.

77. Sally is one of your patients. She weighs 18 lb. Calculate Sally's fluid needs in ml for a 24-hour period (100 ml/kg per d for first 10 kg; 50 ml/kg per d for next 10 kg; and 20 ml/kg per d for any additional kg).

78. The reference dose of pseudoephedrine HCl for children is 4 mg/kg per d PO q.i.d. Available is Novafed syrup 15 mg/5 ml. Calculate the number of tsp/dose for Cynthia, who weighs 35 lb.

79. Clarithromycin is given at 15 mg/kg per d PO b.i.d. Available is Biaxin 125 mg/5 ml. Calculate the number of ml/dose for Dora, who weighs 30 lb.

80. Augmentin 125 mg/ml 1 tsp PO t.i.d. for 10 d is ordered for Alicia. Please interpret this order for Alicia's anxious mom.

81. An ibuprofen reference dose is 20 mg/kg per d PO q8hr p.r.n. fever. Jennifer weighs 38 lb. Calculate the number of ml/dose of the available ibuprofen suspension, 100 mg/5 ml, you should give to Jennifer.

82. Little Rita weighs 36 lb. The reference dose for Septra (trimethoprim; sulfamethoxazole) suspension is 1 tsp/22 lb per dose PO b.i.d. for 10 days. Calculate tsp/dose for Rita.

83. Mikey weighs 44 lb. His doctor ordered ampicillin 100 mg/kg per d. Ampicillin is given PO q.i.d. Calculate mg/dose of ampicillin for Mikey.

84. Molly weighs 11 lb. The recommended fluid administration schedule is as follows: 100 cc/kg per d for the first 10 kg; 50 cc/kg per d for the second 10 kg; then 20 cc/kg per d for each additional kg over 20 kg. What is Molly's fluid requirement over a 12-hr shift?

85. A new mother and her baby are in the clinic for a routine growth and developmental physical examination. The infant is 4 months old and weighs 14 lb 5 oz. The child is taking Enfamil 20 with Iron (20 kcal/fl oz). Based on the reference caloric need for premature infants and infants less than 6 months of age, the appropriate intake is 140 to 150 kcal/kg per d, mom is worried that baby is not taking enough formula.

    a. Calculate the caloric needs of the baby and explain them to this mom.

    b. Calculate the number of fl oz of Enfamil 20/d.

    c. Is the baby receiving a sufficient amount of fluid/d?

    d. Would you recommend a formula with a higher calorie/unit content?

86. The recommended dosage schedule of Tylenol for infants aged 0 to 3 months is 4 mg/kg per dose. Available is Tylenol Infants' Drops 80 mg/0.8 ml. Little Marissa, who is 3 months old, weighs 13 lb. Calculate ml/dose of Tylenol.

87. Ignacio, who is 2½ years old and weighs 40 lb, is transferred to your unit from the emergency department. He is diagnosed with asthma. A theophylline loading dose of 6 mg/kg per d given PO b.i.d. has been ordered. Available is theophylline liquid 80 mg/15 ml. Calculate the tsp/dose of theophylline for Ignacio.

88. The dosage of Septra (trimethoprim; sulfamethoxazole) suspension 1 tsp/22 lb per dose PO b.i.d. Kristen weighs 52 lb. Calculate the number of ml/dose she should receive.

89. The dosage protocol for giving Tylenol elixir (elix) is 1 gr/yr PO q4hr p.r.n. Little Audra is 24 months old. Available is Children's Tylenol elix 160 mg/tsp. Calculate the number of tsp/dose.

90. The reference dose for amoxicillin trihydrate is 40 mg/kg per d PO t.i.d. Luis, who is 7 years old and weighs 52 lb, will take his medication only in liquid form. Available is amoxicillin 250 mg/5 ml.

   a. Calculate the number of mg of amoxicillin/dose for Luis.

   b. Given a choice of ml or tsp, which would you use to administer this dosage?

91. Phenergan with Dextromethorphan (DM) elixir contains promethazine 6.25 mg, and dextromethorphan hydrobromide 15 mg/5 ml. The order for Jim's cough is Phenergan with DM ½ tsp PO q.i.d. p.r.n.

   a. Calculate the number of mg/dose of promethazine.

   b. Calculate the number of mg/dose of dextromethorphan.

92. The order to relieve Mary's pain is morphine 20 μg/kg per hr continuous IV infusion. Mary weighs 42 lb. Calculate the number of mg of morphine/hr.

93. For nausea and vomiting, Phenergan 0.5 mg/kg IM is ordered for Lori, who weighs 28 lb. The available ampule contains Phenergan 25 mg/ml. Calculate the correct number of ml/dose.

94. The reference dose of ampicillin is 100 mg/kg per d IVPB q6hr (infants 1 to 3 months old). Baby Anne, a 6-week-old infant, weighs 9 lb 14 oz. Calculate the number of mg of ampicillin/dose.

95. The Lioresal (baclofen) dose ordered for Larry has been increased to 60 mg/d crushed via NG tube t.i.d. Available is baclofen 5-mg tab. Calculate the number of tab/dose.

96. The reference dose range for ceftriaxone is 50 to 75 mg/kg per d IM (maximum 4 gm/d). Your patient, Tom, is 16 years old and weighs 156 lb. Calculate the dosage range for this patient.

97. The order for Rocephin (ceftriaxone sodium) reads: Rocephin 125 mg IM stat. Available is Rocephin 250 mg sterile crystalline powder in glass vials. To reconstitute for IM administration, the directions call for 0.9 ml of lidocaine (without epinephrine) to make 1 ml of solution. How much of the reconstituted Rocephin will you need to draw up for this order?

98. The gentamicin dosage for patients between 5 and 10 years of age is 6 mg/kg per d IV q8hr. Calculate the number of mg of gentamicin/dose for Jane, an 8-year-old girl who weighs 56 lb.

99. The order of amikacin sulfate for a full-term 7-day-old neonate diagnosed with meningitis reads 2.5 mg/kg per dose IV q8hr. Calculate the number of mg/dose for Baby Roy, who weighs 7 lb 4 oz.

100. Dexamethasone 0.15 mg/kg per dose IV q6hr × 4 d is ordered for Lacey, a 10-month-old infant who weighs 18 lb 10 oz. Available is 4 mg/ml. Calculate the number of ml of dexamethasone/dose.

101. Rose is 9 years old and weighs 67.5 lb. The reference dose for erythromycin stearate is 20 mg/kg per dose q.i.d. Available is erythromycin stearate 200 mg/5 ml. Calculate the number of tsp of erythromycin/dose for Rose.

102. John is to receive 25 mg of Phenergan IM stat. Available is Phenergan in 50-mg/ml ampules. Calculate the number of ml/dose.

103. Unlike erythromycin stearate, the dosage for erythromycin estolate is 30 to 50 mg/kg per d PO q.i.d. Robert is 6 years old and weighs 58 lb. Available is erythromycin estolate suspension 250 mg/5 ml. Calculate the dosage range for Robert in ml/dose.

104. The dosage for isoniazid is 10 mg/kg per d PO q.d. (max 300 mg/d). How much will the child need to weigh in order to receive the maximum dosage of 300 mg/d?

105. Sally, a teenager who weighs 147 lb, is to receive a medication at a rate of 8 μg/kg per min. The medication is in a concentration of 40 mg/250 ml. How long (hr and min) will it take to infuse this medication?

106. Isoniazid can be dosed on a biweekly schedule (2 times/wk), at 20 to 40 mg/kg per dose (max 900 mg/dose). Nancy, who is 12 years old, weighs 116 lb. Calculate the number of mg/biweekly dose.

107. Emma is to receive an initial insulin dose for hyperglycemia and ketonuria. The order reads: Regular Insulin 0.1 U/kg SQ q.i.d. Emma, a 15-year-old girl, weighs 98 lb. How many units of Regular Insulin will Emma receive at each dose?

108. The maximum range for pyrazinamide (PZA) is 2000 mg/d. If the dosage is set at 20 to 30 mg/kg per d, what does the patient need to weigh to receive the maximum dosage?

---

1. Amoxil 2 cap 3 times/d
3. 2 tab/d
5. 18-d supply of Hytrin
7. a. 8 tab/24 hr
   b. Four packages to complete a 14-d regimen
9. 15 dose/5-ml bottle
11. Sustained-release (SR) tab or cap cannot be cut or crushed. Call the pharmacist for a different dosage form.
13. 3 tab/dose
15. She will need to take either 2 tablespoons (tbs) or 6 teaspoons (tsp) of Mylanta to equal the dosage administered in the hospital.

17. 3 tab/d
19. 0.6 ml/dose
21. 28 tab to complete his 2-wk treatment regimen
23. 2 tab/dose
25. a. 50.5 = 51 ml of stock ETOH
    b. 480 − 51 ml = 429 ml
    c. 9.4 pt of 10% ETOH. If you round down and use 50 ml/pt, you get 9.6 ml. In reality, you would most likely mix 1 pt of stock solution with 9 pt of water to make this solution.
27. 0.53 ml/dose
29. 0.15 ml/dose

31. 4 vials
33. 0.95 = 1 ml/dose
35. 200 mg/ml
37. 10.5 = 11 μgtt/min
39. 3.2 ml
41. 360 kcal/d
43. a. 2.4 kg
    b. 7.3 = 7 μgtt/min
45. 4 ml/dose
47. 3.75 ml/bolus dose
49. a. Add 0.42 ml of Decadron to 50 ml of D_5W solution.
    b. 37.5 = 38 gtt/min
51. 25 gtt/min
53. a. 125 gtt/min bolus dose
    b. 10.4 = 10 gtt/min KVO
55. a. Add 9.6 ml of NaCl to 500 ml of D_5W.
    b. Add 5 ml of KCl to 500 ml of D_5W with NaCl.
57. a. Add 8.2 ml of aminophylline to 100 ml of D_5W.
    b. 75 gtt/min
59. 350 ml
61. Add 6.2 ml of Hydrocortone Phosphate to the 50-ml NS unit bag.
63. a. 2 vial/dose
    b. 25 gtt/min
65. a. 5.6 ml of diluent per 2 gm of Cefobid
    b. 100 ml of NS per 2 gm of Cefobid
    c. 200 ml/hr
67. 50 gtt/min

69. You will need to place a new bag in about 56 min (6:56 AM)
71. 13.2 = 13 ml/hr
73. 25 ml/hr
75. 0.3 mg/dose
77. 818 ml/d (820 ml/d)
79. 4 ml/dose
81. 5.8 = 6 ml/dose. It is difficult to measure 0.8 of a ml using a standard PO delivery system, such as tsp or dropper.
83. 500 mg/dose
85. a. 911 to 976 kcal/d
    b. 45 to 49 fl oz/d
    c. The baby needs only 650 ml/d; however, the baby is consuming between 1350 and 1470 ml/d in formula, an *excess* of 700 to 820 ml/d.
    d. Yes, a higher caloric content is very appropriate, i.e., 30 kcal/fl oz.
87. 2 tsp/dose
89. 0.75 = ¾ tsp/dose
91. a. 3.1 mg promethazine/dose
    b. 7.5 mg dextromethorphan/dose
93. 0.25 ml/dose
95. 4 tab/dose
97. 0.5 ml/dose
99. 8.2 mg/dose
101. 3 tsp/dose
103. 4 ml to 6.6 ml/dose
105. 74.8 min = 1 hr and 15 min
107. 4.5 U/dose

Bibliography

Albert GA. Medication errors: A disciplinary approach to prevention for nurses. Neonatal Pharmacol Q 2:37–42, 1993.

Arndt M. Nurses' medication errors. J Adv Nurs 19:519–526, 1994.

Arnold L. Our safety is important too. Am J Nurs 97:80, 1997.

Baer CL, Williams BR. Clinical Pharmacology and Nursing, 2nd ed. Springhouse, PA, Springhouse Corp, 1992.

Barnhart ER. Physician's Desk Reference (PDR), 49th ed. Oradel, NJ, Medical Economics Co, 1996.

Bayne T, Bindler R. Medication calculation skills of registered nurses. J Contin Educ Nurs 19:258–262, 1988.

Bindler B, Bayne T. Do baccalaureate students possess basic mathematics proficiency? J Nurs Educ 23:192–197, 1984.

Bindler B, Bayne T. Medication calculation ability of registered nurses. Image J Nurs Sch 23:221–224, 1991.

Bliss-Holtz J. Discriminating types of medication calculation errors in nursing practice. Nurs Res 43:373–375, 1994.

Booker MF, Ignatavicius DD. Infusion Therapy Techniques & Medications, Philadelphia, WB Saunders Co, 1996.

Carlisle D. Just one slip: Penalized for a mistake in drug administration. Nurs Times 87:30–31, 1994.

Chan PD, Safani M. Physicians' Drug Resource with Dosage, Side Effect, and Drug Interaction, and All Newly Approved Drugs. Fountain Valley, CA, Current Clinical Strategies, 1996.

Chan PD, Winkle PJ, Winkle CR. Family Medicine, 2nd ed. Fountain Valley, CA, Current Clinical Strategies, 1995.

Cohen MR. Taking this test will help you avoid errors. Nursing 20:23–24, 1991.

Cooper MC. Can a zero defect philosophy be applied to drug errors? J Adv Nurs 21:487–491, 1995.

Craig GP, Sellers SC. The effects of dimensional analysis on the medication dosage calculation abilities of nursing students. Nurse Educ 20:14–18, 1995.

Current Pediatric Diagnosis and Treatment. Hay WW, Groothuis JR, Hayward AR, et al, eds. Norwalk, CT, Appleton & Lange, 1995.

Davis NM. Teaching patients to prevent errors. Am J Nurs 94:17, 1994.

DelGaudio D, Menonna-Quinn D. Chemotherapy: Potential occupational hazards. Am J Nurs 98:59–65, 1998.

Doucette LJ. Mathematics for the Clinical Laboratory, Philadelphia, WB Saunders Co, 1997.

Fink J. Preventing lawsuits: Medication errors to avoid. Nurs Life 3:26–29, 1983.

Gennrich JL, Chan PD. Pediatric Drug Reference with Dosage, Side Effect, and Drug Interaction Comments. Fountain Valley, CA, Current Clinical Strategies, 1996.

Gillespie JL. Five things you should know about medicine cabinets: Teach your patient how to store medications properly— before they're ruined. Nursing 25:13, 1995.

Goodstein M. Reflections upon mathematics in the introductory chemistry course. J Chem Educ 60:665–667, 1983.

The Harriet Lane Handbook: A Manual for Pediatric House Officers, 14th ed. Michael A. Barone, ed. St. Louis, CV Mosby Co, 1996.

Harrison's Principles of Internal Medicine, Vol 1 & 2, 12th ed. Braunwald E et al, eds. New York, McGraw-Hill, Inc, 1991.

Herrman F. Four kinds of carelessness that can send you to court. Nurs Life 2:63, 1982.

Joiner GA. Developing a proactive approach to medication error prevention. J Healthcare Qual 16:35–40, 1994.

Kelly LY. The Nursing Experience: Trends, Challenges, and Transitions, 2nd ed. New York, McGraw-Hill, Inc, 1992.

Killian WH. Medication errors expose RNs to liability. Am Nurse 23:34, 1991.

Koska MT. Teaching hospitals to track, prevent drug errors. Hospitals 66:69–70, 1991.

Leff L. Survey of math, science skills puts U.S. students at the bottom. Washington Post, February 1, 1989, A14, A16.

Lilley LL, Guanci R. Careful with zeroes. Am J Nurs 97:14, 1997.

Lilley LL, Guanci R. When 'look-alikes' and 'sound-alikes' don't act alike. Am J Nurs 97:12, 14, 1997.

Lilley LL, Guanci R. Look-alike abbreviations: Prescriptions for confusion. Am J Nurs 97:12, 14, 1997.

Loebel AB. Chemical Problem-Solving by Dimensional Analysis: A Self-Instructional Program, 3rd ed. Boston, Houghton Mifflin Co, 1987.

Martin PJ. Professional updating through open learning as a method of reducing errors in the administration of medicine. J Nurs Manage 2:209–212, 1994.

McClure ML. Human error: A professional dilemma. J Prof Nurs 7:207, 1991.

Miller-Keane Encyclopedia and Dictionary of Medicine, Nursing, and Allied Health, 6th ed. O'Toole MR, ed. Philadelphia, WB Saunders Co, 1997.

Northrop C, Kelly M: Legal Issues in Nursing. St. Louis, CV Mosby Co, 1987.

Pinnell, JL: Nursing Pharmacology. Philadelphia, WB Saunders Co, 1996.

Roseman C, Booker JM. Workload and environmental factors in hospital medication errors. Nurs Res 44:226–230, 1995.

Scholz DA. Establishing and monitoring an endemic medication error rate. J Nurs Qual Assur 4:71–74, 1990.

Senders JW. Detecting, correcting, and interrupting errors. J Intravenous Nurs 18:28–32, 1995.

Simonsen LLP. Top 200 drugs Rx prices still moderating as managed care grows. Pharmacy Times, April, 17–23, 1995.

Slattery M. The epidemic hazards of nursing. Am J Nurs 98:50–53, 1998.

Smith LS. Those medication error dilemmas! Adv Clin Care 5:50–51, 1990.

Spradley BW. Community Health Nursing Concepts and Practice, 3rd ed. Glenview, IL, Scott, Foresman & Co, 1990.

Spradley BW, & Allender JA. Community Health Nursing: Concepts & Practice. 4th ed. Philadelphia, Lippincott-Raven, 1996.

Taber's Cyclopedic Medical Dictionary, Thomas CL, ed. 16 ed. Philadelphia, FA Davis Co, 1992.

Thigpen J. Education in the NICU. Minimizing medication errors. Neonatal Network 14:85–86, 1995.

Vonfrolio LG, Noone J. The Emergency Nursing Examination Review, 2nd ed. Springhouse, PA, Springhouse Corp, 1991.

Wolf ZR. Medication errors and nursing responsibility. Holistic Nurs Pract 4:8–17, 1989.

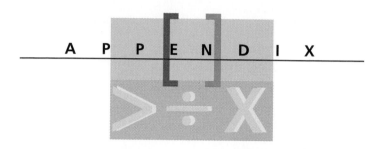

INTRODUCTION TO THE SYSTEMS OF MEASUREMENT

Medications can be categorized according to their physical states or dimensions, that is, how they exist in nature. As in nature, medications come in solid, liquid, and gaseous forms. A good way of deciding whether a medication is solid or not is by figuring out whether it flows. A simple rule: Any medication that can be poured is best measured by its volume. Therefore, medications that flow come labeled with dimensional units pertaining to volume, such as ml, tsp, gtt, or fl oz.

What if the medication does not flow? In order to measure nonflowing medications, you may need to count, weigh, measure, or calculate their dimensions. So, as a rule, you can safely measure solids by their dimensions and weight, and liquids and gases by their volume. In instances involving distances, you will measure the medications by their linear dimension.

The three systems of measurement used in dosage calculation are the metric system, the US customary system of measurement, and the English system. Most medications come in metric units. Nevertheless, in dosage administration, both systems are used quite often. Therefore, to move from one to another, we need to know the equivalencies of the unit systems.

Metric System

The metric system uses a series of unit prefixes for weight, volume, and linear measurements. These units are interchangeable by a factor of 10 in moving from one layer of standardized prefixes to the next. The prefixes are then tagged with physical state units, for example, gram for weight; liter for volume, meter for linear measurement; bel for sound; joule for energy, watt for power.

 Memorize the prefix units of the metric system.

 You are able to convert "kilo-" to "milli-" by moving the decimal point.

Metric units from the largest to the smallest:

Prefix Unit (Symbols)	Weight (Symbols) -gram	Volume (Symbols) -liter	Linear (Symbols) -meter	Equivalency Factor to Standard Unit (Factorial)
kilo- (k)	kilogram (kg)		kilometer (km)	0.001 (1×10^{-3})
hecto- (h)	hectogram (hg)		hectometer (hm)	0.01 (1×10^{-2})
deka- (dk)	dekagram (dkg)		dekameter (dkm)	0.1 (1×10^{-1})
Standard Unit	gram (g)	liter (L)	meter (m)	1.0
deci- (d)	decigram (dg)	deciliter (dl)	decimeter (dm)	10.0 (1×10^{1})
centi- (c)	centigram (cg)	centiliter (cl)	centimeter (cm)	100.0 (1×10^{2})
milli- (m)	milligram (mg)	milliliter (ml)	millimeter (mm)	1,000.0 (1×10^{3})
micro- (μ)	microgram (μg)	microliter (μl)	micrometer (μm)	1,000,000.0 (1×10^{6})
nano- (n)	nanogram (ng)	nanoliter (nl)	nanometer (nm)	1,000,000,000.0 (1×10^{9})
pico- (p)	picogram (pg)	picoliter (pl)	picometer (pm)	(1×10^{12})

NOTES

English System or the US Customary System

1. Apothecaries' Weight and Avoirdupois Weight

These are the oldest systems of weight measurement.

Apothecaries' Weight	Avoirdupois Weight
12 ounces (oz) = 1 pound (lb)	16 ounces (oz) = 1 pound (lb) 2000 pounds (lb) = 1 short ton

2. US Customary System of Volume Measurement

These measurements may look familiar to you. You will find these in all American recipes and cookbooks.

4 microdrops (μgtt)	=	1 drop (gtt)
1 drop (gtt)	=	1 minim (m)
1 teaspoon (tsp)	=	1 fluid dram (fl dr)
3 teaspoons (tsp)	=	1 tablespoon (tbsp)
2 tablespoons (tbsp)	=	1 fluid ounce (fl oz)
6 fluid ounces (fl oz)	=	1 teacup (tc)
8 fluid ounces (fl oz)	=	1 measuring cup (c)
2 measuring cups (c)	=	1 pint (pt)
2 pints (pt)	=	1 quart (qt)
4 quarts (qt)	=	1 gallon (gal)

UNIT EQUIVALENCE TABLES

The following table contains some common metric and nonmetric conversion equivalencies. Using this table, the units provided under the metric and nonmetric sections, and dimensional analysis (DA), you will be able to convert one system to another without difficulty.

Weight Equivalents

This table gives you quite a few unit equivalencies between metric and nonmetric systems. You will definitely use some of these equivalencies, but not all of them.

Metric Measure	US Customary Measure
60–65 mg	= 1 gr
1 gm	= 15.43 gr (15–16 gr)
1 gm	= 0.353 oz
30 gm	= 2 tbsp
1 kg	= 2.2 lb

Volume Equivalents

The table below serves as a good reference for volume equivalencies.

Metric Measure	US Customary Measure	
0.06–0.07 ml	= 1 gtt	= 1 minim (m)
1 ml	= 15–16 gtt	= 15–16 m
1 ml	= 60 μgtt	
4–5 ml	= 1 tsp	= 1 fl dram (dr)
15–16 ml	= 1 tbsp	= 4 fl dram (dr)
30–32 ml	= 2 tbsp	
30–32 ml	= 1 fl oz	
240–250 ml	= 1 measuring cup (c)	
473.1765 ml	= 1 pt	
1000 ml	= 1.0567 qt	
3785 ml	= 1 gal	

Distance Equivalents

The two pertinent linear unit equivalencies will be inch/foot (ft), and centimeter (cm)/inch.

$$12 \text{ inches} = 1 \text{ foot}$$

$$2.54 \text{ centimeters} = 1 \text{ inch}$$

Time Units

The following table lists time units and their unit equivalencies.

60 seconds (sec)	=	1 minute (min)
60 minutes (min)	=	1 hour (hr)
24 hours (hr)	=	1 day (d)

Temperature Conversion

From Celsius (Centigrade) to Fahrenheit:

$$(°C \times \tfrac{9}{5}) + 32 = °F$$

EXAMPLE 1

Convert 38° Celsius to Fahrenheit.

$$38°C \times \tfrac{9}{5} + 32 = 100.4°F$$

1. Multiply 38 by 9 = 342
2. Divide 342 by 5 = 68.4
3. Add 32 to 68.4 = 100.4

From Fahrenheit to Celsius:

$$(°F - 32) \times \tfrac{5}{9} = °C$$

EXAMPLE 2

Convert 101°F to Celsius.

$$(101°F - 32) \times \tfrac{5}{9} = 38.3°C$$

1. Subtract 32 from 101 = 69
2. Multiply 69 by 5 = 345
3. Divide 345 by 9 = 38.3

ABBREVIATIONS IN LATIN AND ENGLISH

The effective use of abbreviations saves a lot of time; however, both the writer and the reader have to recognize and interpret the abbreviation correctly. Therefore, you will need to be proficient in interpreting abbreviations that are commonly found on patients' charts and/or given in medication dosage orders. The following table provides most of the abbreviations frequently used in medication dosage orders.

Abbreviation	Latin	English
a	*ante*	before
aa		so much of each
AA		amino acid
a.c.	*ante cibum*	before meal
AC		alternating current
ad lib.	*ad libitum*	as desired
agit.	*agita*	shake
alb.	*albus*	white
aq.	*aqua*	water
b.i.d.	*bis in die*	twice daily
bis in 7 d.	*bis in septem diebus*	twice a week
BM		bowel movement
BP		blood pressure
c.	*cum*	with

Abbreviation	Latin	English
C		Celsius
		Centigrade
c		cup
CAD		coronary artery disease
cal		calorie
cap		capsule, caplet
cc		cubic centimeter
CC		chief complaint
Cl		chloride
cm		centimeter
CVA		cerebrovascular accident
d.	*dexter*	right
	dies	day
DC		discharge
		direct current
dc		discontinue
decub.	*decubitus*	lying down
dil.	*dilue*	dilute or dissolve
dl		deciliter
DM		diabetes mellitus
DT		diphtheria and tetanus [toxoid]
DTP		diphtheria, tetanus toxoids, and pertussis [vaccine]
D_5W		dextrose 5% in water
Dx		diagnosis
Dz		disease
ED		emergency department
elix		elixir
ER		emergency room
ETA		endotracheal airway
ext		extract
F		Fahrenheit
fl oz		fluid ounce
fru.		fructose
g		gram
GLU		glucose
gm		gram
gr		grain
gtt	*guttae*	drops
h.	*hora*	hour
H		hypodermic
		hydrogen
HCl		hydrochloride
HCO_3^-		bicarbonate ion
HCTZ		hydrochlorothiazide
Hep B		hepatitis B vaccine
Hib		*Haemophilus influenzae* b vaccine
h.s.	*hora somni*	at bedtime
ht		height
HTN		hypertension
IM		intramuscularly
inf.	*infusum*	infusion
INH		isoniazid
inhal.	*inhalatio*	inhalation
inj.	*injectio*	injection
IT		intrathecally
IU		International Unit
IV		intravenously

Abbreviation	Latin	English
IVPB		intravenous piggyback
IVSP		intravenous slow push
kcal		kilocalorie
KCl		potassium chloride
kg		kilogram
KVO		keep vein open
L		liter
lb		pound
LD_{50}		median lethal dose
liq.	*liquor*	liquid
lot.	*lotio*	lotion
LR		lactated Ringer's solution
m		meter
mEq		milliequivalent
μg		microgram
mg		milligram
μgtt		microdrop
min		minute
ml		milliliter
mm		millimeter
MMR		measles, mumps, rubella [vaccine]
MOM		milk of magnesia
mU		milliunit
NaCl		sodium chloride
NAD		no acute distress
$NaHCO_3$		sodium bicarbonate
npo	*nil per os*	nothing by mouth
NS		normal saline
O.D.	*oculus dexter*	right eye
O.S.	*oculus sinister*	left eye
O.U.	*oculus uterque*	each eye
oz		ounce
p	*post*	after
p.c.	*post cibum*	after meal
PERRL		pupils equal, regular, react to light
PI		present illness
PMH		past medical history
PMS		premenstrual syndrome
PO	*per os*	by mouth
PO_4		phosphate
PPD		purified protein derivative [tuberculin test]
PR	*per rectum*	by way of the rectum
p.r.n.	*pro re nata*	as needed
PV	*per vaginam*	through the vagina
pt		pint
q2hr		every 2 hours
q3hr		every 3 hours
q.d.	*quaque die*	every day
q.h.	*quaque hora*	every hour
q.i.d.	*quater in die*	four times daily
Rx		prescription
		take
s.	*sine*	without
S		sulfur
sec		second
SC	*sub cutis*	subcutaneously
SO_4		sulfate
sol.	*solutio*	solution

Abbreviation	Latin	English
S/P	*status post*	no change after
SQ		subcutaneously
ss.	*semis*	half
stat	*statim*	immediately
supp	*suppositorium*	suppository
syr.	*syrupus*	syrup
tab	*tabella*	tablet
tbsp		tablespoon
t.i.d.	*ter in die*	three times a day
t.i.n.	*ter in nocte*	three times a night
tinct.	*tinctura*	tincture
top		topical
TPR		temperature, pulse, respiration
tsp		teaspoon
U		unit
ung.	*unguentum*	ointment
UV		ultraviolet
vit		vitamin
WA		while awake
wk		week
wt		weight
y/o		year(s) old
yr		year

NOMOGRAM FOR BODY SURFACE AREA

To calculate medication dosages based on the patient's body surface area (BSA), you will need to refer to a nomogram. A nomogram is a calibrated scale that correlates growth, that is, heights (using inches or cm), and body weight (measured in lb or kg) of a population (adults and/or children). You can follow the steps provided to determine your patient's BSA.

1. Find the weight of your patient (lb or kg) on the weight line (the vertical line farthest to the right).
2. Find the height of your patient (cm or inches) on the height line (the vertical line farthest to the left).
3. Take a transparent ruler and plot a line between those two points.
4. The surface area of your patient (m^2) will be where your ruler intersects the surface area line (the vertical line in the middle between the height and the weight lines).

Most adult BSA values are approximately equal to 1.73 m^2.

RECOMMENDED IMMUNIZATION SCHEDULE FOR INFANTS AND CHILDREN

The following table lists the immunizations and a schedule for their administration as recommended by the American Pediatric Association. An additional schedule needs to be consulted for infants and children who do not follow the schedule as recommended, for example, late-starters, immigrants, those receiving boosters.

	Birth to 1 mo	1 mo	2 mo	4 mo	6 mo	12 mo	15 to 18 mo	4 to 6 yr
OPV*			✓	✓	✓			✓
DTP†			✓	✓	✓		✓	✓
Hib			✓	✓	✓		✓	
MMR						✓		✓
HepB	✓	✓			✓			
VariVax‡						✓		

*First and second dose OPV may use inactivated poliomyelitis vaccine (IPV) instead.
†Dtap instead of DTP may be given.
‡VariVax after age 1 yr.

To find the body surface area, locate the height in inches (or centimeters) on scale I and the weight in pounds (or kilograms) on scale III. A straight-edged ruler placed between those two points will intersect scale II and determine the client's surface area. (From DuBois, E. F. [1936]. Basal metabolism in health and disease. Philadelphia: Lea & Febiger. Copyright 1920 by W. M. Boothby and R. B. Sandiford.)

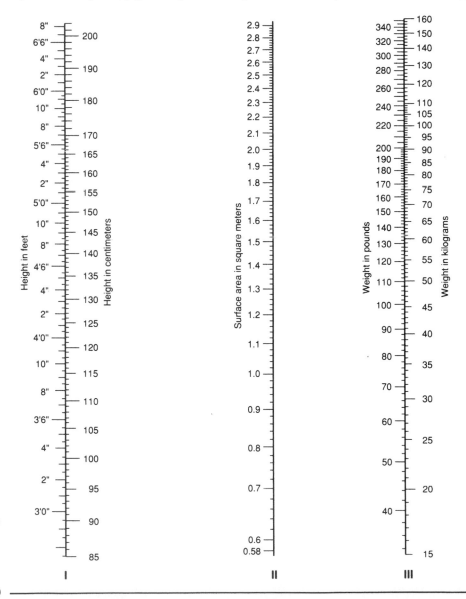

Figure 1. *Dubois' body surface area chart. (From O'Toole MR, ed.* Miller-Keane Encyclopedia and Dictionary of Medicine, Nursing and Allied Health *6th ed. Philadelphia, WB Saunders, 1997, p. 1840, with permission.)*

PATIENT'S BILL OF RIGHTS: THE RIGHT TO REFUSE TREATMENT

The fourth article under a Patient's Bill of Rights addresses the right of the patient to refuse treatment. In addition to the American Hospital Association's guideline on the patient's bill of rights, each institution may implement additional articles of patients' rights according to that institution's philosophy.

1. The patient has the right to considerate and respectful care.
2. The patient has the right to obtain from his physician complete current information concerning his diagnosis, treatment, and prognosis, in terms the patient can be reasonably expected to understand. When it is not medically advisable to give such information to the patient, the information should be made available to an appropriate person in his behalf. He has the right to know by name the physician responsible for coordinating his care.
3. The patient has the right to receive from his physician information necessary to give informed consent prior to the start of any procedure and/or treatment. Except in emergencies, such information for informed consent should include but not necessarily be limited to the specific procedure and/or treatment, the medically significant risks involved, and the probable duration of incapacitation. Where medically significant alternatives for care or treatment exist, or when the patient requests information concerning medical alternatives, the patient has the right to such information. The patient also has the right to know the name of the person responsible for the procedures and/or treatment.
4. The patient has the right to refuse treatment to the extent permitted by law and to be informed of the medical consequences of his action.
5. The patient has the right to every consideration of his privacy concerning his own medical care program. Case discussion, consultation, examination, and treatment are confidential and should be conducted discreetly. Those not directly involved in this care must have the permission of the patient to be present.
6. The patient has the right to expect that all communications and records pertaining to his care should be treated as confidential.
7. The patient has the right to expect that within its capacity, a hospital must make reasonable response to the request of a patient for services. The hospital must provide evaluation, service, and/or referral as indicated by the urgency of the case. When medically permissible, a patient may be transferred to another facility only after he has received complete information and explanation concerning the needs for and alternatives to such a transfer. The institution to which the patient is transferred must first have accepted the patient for transfer.
8. The patient has the right to obtain information as to any relationship of his hospital to other health care and educational institutions insofar as his care is concerned. The patient has the right to obtain information as to the existence of any professional relationships among individuals, by name, who are treating him.
9. The patient has the right to be advised if the hospital proposes to engage in or perform human experimentation affecting his care or treatment. The patient has the right to refuse to participate in such research projects.
10. The patient has the right to expect reasonable continuity of care. He has the right to know in advance what appointment times and physicians are available and where. The patient has the right to expect that the hospital will provide a mechanism whereby he is informed by his physician or a delegate of the physician of the patient's continuing health.
11. The patient has the right to examine and receive an explanation of his bill regardless of source of payment.
12. The patient has the right to know what hospital rules and regulations apply to his conduct as a patient.

Source: American Hospital Association, 1973. A patient's bill of rights, *Nursing Outlook,* February 1973, 21:82, and January 1976, 24:29.

NEEDLE AND SYRINGES

Needles vary in gauge (the width of the bore) and length. The larger the gauge, the smaller the bore. Needle lengths vary from $\frac{3}{8}$ inch to 3 inches Syringes vary according to the volume they measure.

The calibration marks on a syringe decrease in precision as the syringe size increases. The smaller the syringe, the more accurately you can measure volume, for example, to the 100th of a ml with a 1-ml syringe (tuberculin). The following illustrations display the components of needles and syringes.

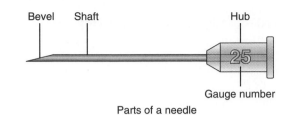

Bevel   Shaft   Hub

Gauge number

Parts of a needle

Figure 2. *Components of syringe and needle. (From Leahy JM, Kizilay PE, eds.* Foundations of Nursing Practice: A Nursing Process Approach. *Philadelphia, WB Saunders, 1998, p. 469, with permission.)*

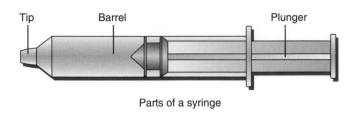

Tip   Barrel   Plunger

Parts of a syringe

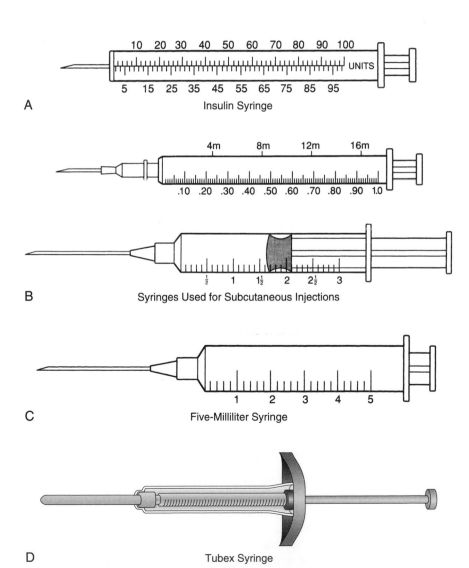

A   Insulin Syringe

B   Syringes Used for Subcutaneous Injections

C   Five-Milliliter Syringe

Figure 3. A *to* D, *Types of syringes. (*A *to* C *From Kee JL, Marshall SM, eds.* Clinical Calculations *2nd ed. Philadelphia, WB Saunders, 1992, pp. 97, 98.* D *Modified from Leahy JM, Kizilay PB, eds.* Foundations of Nursing Practice: A Nursing Process Approach. *Philadelphia, WB Saunders, 1998, p. 469, with permission.)*

D   Tubex Syringe

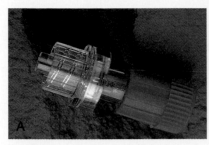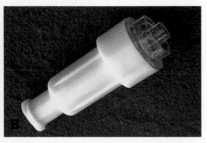

Figure 4. *Needleless administration system, ports.* A, *SafSite® valve and "deadhead."* B, *Ultrasite® syringe. (Courtesy of B. Braun Medical, Inc., Bethlehem, PA.)*

The implementation of needleless systems increases occupational safety in the prevention of needle-stick injuries. You need to check the ports for markings that distinctly differentiate needleless systems from conventional ports.

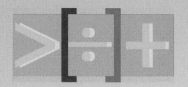

Index

Page numbers in *italics* refer to illustrations; page numbers followed by t refer to tables.

A

B

C

D